TAKE TWO APPLES AND
CALL ME IN THE MORNING

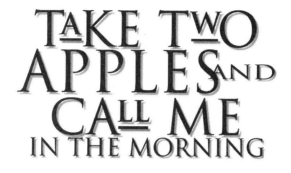

TAKE TWO APPLES AND CALL ME IN THE MORNING

JUDY STONE

CN, M.S.W.

HARA
PUBLISHING GROUP

TAKE TWO APPLES AND
CALL ME IN THE MORNING

Published by

Hara Publishing · P.O. Box 19732 · Seattle, WA 98109

© 2003 by Judy Stone

All rights reserved

ISBN 1-883697-48-4
Library of Congress Control Number 2002101806

Editor: Victoria McCown
Book Design and Cover by Robilyn Robbins
Indexer: Judith Gibbs
Cover Photograph: ©elektraVision AG/PictureQuest ©2000

Printed in the United States of America

Stone, Judy.
   Take two apples and call me in the morning / Judy
Stone. -- 1st ed.
      p. cm.
   Includes bibliographical references and index.
   LCCN 1-883697-48-4

   1. Nutrition--Popular works. 2. Health   I. Title

RA784.S76 2002   613.2
                        QBI33-698

IN MEMORY

of my father, Stephen Stone,

whose compassion, integrity, and reflection

continue to light my way.

CONTENTS

ACKNOWLEDGEMENTS

Oftentimes the best recipe is one in which many undetectable ingredients combine to give the finished product its full flavor. So it was with the writing of this book. My list of secret ingredients includes Deborah Stone, who has always been my inspiration, chief supporter, cooking companion, and a most fabulous sister. My mom emphasized the importance of chocolate in any well-balanced diet, set a great example of creativity with food, and had the courage to give me free rein in the kitchen at a very early age. My dad had the courage to eat the results, always with great appreciation, though perhaps not always so deserved. He also challenged me, as soon as I was old enough to engage in conversation, to question everything, a trait, as my parent, I'm sure he grew to regret on many occasions!

For over 20 years I have been part of a most incredible group of colleagues whose love, wisdom, and willingness to grow has deepened both my understanding of how we humans change and my faith in our capacity to do so, if given the right support.

My colleague and friend, Rachel Albert-Matesz, has shared most generously her wealth of nutrition and cooking knowledge. Rachel contributed some of my favorite recipes in this book, which will also appear in her book *The Natural Food Plan: A Produce-Dominated Diet and Cookbook* due out in January 2003.

My dear friend and personal trainer, Ann-Margaret Giovino, was my coach and cheerleader throughout the writing of this book, and without her support this book would not have left the recesses of my computer.

I wish to thank Sheryn Hara of Hara Publishing Group in Seattle, editor Vicki McCown, designer Robilyn Robbins, and indexer Judith Gibbs. Once the cooking is done, any meal can be served haphazardly on a plate. A meal that nourishes all our senses is artfully arranged and lovingly presented, and so it was with this book.

PREFACE

The controversy in recent years among government officials, the media, nutritionists, diet gurus, and consumers over the "low-carbohydrate diet" phenomenon is nothing short of a good old-fashioned, lunchroom food fight. Whatever you know or don't know, believe or don't believe about the low-carbohydrate trend, no one disagrees with the fact that the predominance of overly processed carbohydrates, sugar, fast food, and highly manufactured products has spawned a health crisis of great magnitude in this country. It would be hard to make a case otherwise when we look at the epidemic occurrence of diabetes, obesity, ADD/ADHD, depression, high cholesterol, hypertension, and other chronic illnesses.

In my own small corner of the world, practicing as both a psychotherapist and a nutritionist, I have been awed by the power of food to change people's lives. Significantly reducing their consumption of sugar and refined carbohydrates has produced nothing short of miracles in many of my clients' lives and in their emotional and physical health. So dramatic were these changes that I began to feel I could do more to help people in less time as a nutritionist than as a psychotherapist, which eventually prompted me to focus my practice solely on nutrition. In addition to nutrition coaching, I also teach cooking classes, present corporate wellness programs, write articles, and give workshops, and the appetite for this information is huge. What I see, though, is that as hungry as people are, all too often the desire of well-intentioned people to improve health gets buried by frustration, confusion, and ambivalence about learning a different way of eating.

We live in a society that makes it cheaper and more convenient to eat poorly. We exist at a time in history when forty years of misguided but persuasive thinking about the role of dietary fat has created a powerful "low-fat economy" based on thousands of products that increase the very problems they claim to prevent. This economy is supported by a pharmaceutical industry eagerly serving up costly drugs to clean up the mess. The bottom line? It's been too difficult and too unappealing for most Americans to give up a way of eating that has been made more affordable, more convenient, in our minds more correct, and in our experience more tasty.

We are a nation of people who have come to rely on experts and magic bullets to lead us into health. Although "experts" can be a wonderful source of inspiration and gathered knowledge, they are no substitute for cultivating our own desires and inner wisdom to guide us through change. And magic bullets don't come cheap. There is and always will be a price we pay for "easy." The price might be in the dollars we pay for medical care, fancy spas, personal chefs, or structured diet programs. Or it will likely be at a more precious price, the cost of our health and quality of life when we use a myriad of medications with all their side effects, or the cost to our well-being and our self esteem when nothing we try works. We've been sold "instant," and that's what we're used to—instant pudding, instant weight loss, instant drug relief. But changing our individually and collectively declining health requires more time and patience than "add milk and stir," "lose ten pounds by Christmas," or "just one pill spells relief."

Many people have gotten the message that 90 percent of illness and poor health can be treated or reversed through daily behavior choices that each of us has under our control, such as food, exercise, drinking, and smoking. After talking over the past few years with hundreds of people about nutrition and health, what I have noticed is that more people than ever are aware of the toxicity of sugar, refined carbohydrates, and manufactured fats. But most are overwhelmed by the prospect of making the shift to a healthier way of eating in the midst of already overburdened lives. It's no wonder we are still choosing to spend billions annually on high-priced drugs, high-tech surgical procedures, and out-of-control health insurance premiums.

My vision for this book was to create a coaching manual that would inform, inspire, and be the next best thing to having a personal nutrition *and* cooking coach available 24/7. Understanding how the body uses the food you're eating to either support or deplete health is a great motivator for you to make a change. But translating that understanding into action is another "kettle of fish," as the saying goes. The gaps between knowing what to do, knowing *how* to do it, and doing it consistently can be quite large, and they have swallowed many of us repeatedly. Learning to tell the difference between what nourishes your body and what fattens the food industry at your expense isn't easy. There are so many other pieces that contribute to long-term health and that can support your efforts to change—things like beliefs and attitudes, exercise, sleep habits, supplements, etc. But trying to "just do it" can send you scurrying in too many directions, getting you nowhere at all.

Take Two Apples and Call Me in the Morning is a meal of many courses, carefully made with all of the ingredients that have been helpful to my clients and students over the years. I serve it to you with the hope that it will inspire in you an enthusiasm to take charge of your health in what I believe is the most powerful and direct way possible—through the food you eat every day. This is an ongoing meal not meant for you to devour in one or two sittings—you will surely feel stuffed and uncomfortable if you approach it that way. It is not a diet program, although it does have concrete suggestions for structuring your eating based on an understanding of *your* body and *your* physical and emotional health needs. This book may not give you the high of the latest, dramatic diet plan. It is grounded in good nutrition, but, more important, it is grounded in the reality of how people like you or I plan for, execute, and integrate big changes that will stick for the long haul. One step at a time. Your time.

I will consider this book successful if your desire to eat differently and exercise regularly is ignited, not because I've convinced you of anything, but because after trying a few small changes, you are not able to ignore how much better you feel. And I will consider it successful if, beyond that, it continues to provide you with the support, information, and guidance you need to keep building on those first delicious experiences of better health.

HOW TO USE THIS BOOK

This book has three purposes. The first is to demystify nutrition by correcting fallacies that have become doctrine in the last few decades and by presenting some of the current thinking in the relationship between what you eat and how you feel. I have pulled from many sources and resources to help you separate the "wheat from the chaff" and to enable you to make informed choices about what you put in your body.

The second is to take judgement, rigidity, frustration, deprivation, and futility out of trying to change how you eat and to replace those with patience, compassion, and reality. *Take Two Apples and Call Me in the Morning* is written to reflect the reality of how real people learn and change. Effective change is not instant and it's rarely ever a continual move in a single direction. Being flexible and compassionate enough to grow at your own pace is a key to success in any endeavor. This book will help you both challenge yourself to set and meet your goals and give you room to be human.

The third purpose of this book is to hold your hand in the kitchen, as much as this print medium allows, until you get comfortable with eating a healthier diet. If you're going to eat healthy food, learning what to buy, where to buy it, and how to prepare it is certainly a necessity. And if you're not a cook, there are chapters and ideas to support your healthy eating as well.

I've structured *Take Two Apples and Call Me in the Morning* to be both informative and practical. The first seven chapters are each divided into three sections: Understanding Your Body, Nutrition Magic, and Moving Forward. In UNDERSTANDING YOUR BODY I present in a clear and simple way how your body and brain work with the food you eat, describing how different foods enhance your well-being or deplete your health. These sections look at how the food that makes up most people's diets—refined carbohydrates, sugar, poor-quality fat, caffeine, and highly manufactured foods—affect emotional and physical health. It also looks at how we have gotten away from eating the food who perceive themselves to be healthy and are simply trying to stay that way find a diet that keeps blood sugar well-regulated gives them more energy, clarity, and emotional well-being.

The *Understanding Your Body* section of Chapter One will teach you how highs and lows in blood sugar are related to many aspects of your health, and to how you feel every day. Next, the concrete suggestions in the *Nutrition Magic* section will lead you into the kitchen and on to the path of feeling better NOW! In the *Moving Forward* section, you'll find some helpful tools for working with your mental readiness for making changes. Taking the time to work with these tools will insure that the changes you are making will firmly take hold and keep you on the path to better health.

UNDERSTANDING YOUR BODY

All the food we eat can be divided into three categories: protein, carbohydrate, and fat. This chapter will focus on carbohydrates and their role in health and disease. We'll get to protein and fat a little bit later.

WHICH FOODS ARE CARBOHYDRATES?

The category of Carbohydrates includes: bread, pasta, cereals (hot and cold), baked goods, soda pop, snack foods, all sweeteners— natural and otherwise—fruits and their juices, vegetables, whole grains, and beans or legumes.

Carbohydrates affect your body and brain differently than either protein or fat. And different kinds of carbohydrates affect your blood sugar regulation and health differently. Exactly how carbohydrates affect your health, and how you feel on a daily basis, is the focus of this chapter. You may have heard a lot of conflicting information in the press, from doctors or nutritionists, or from friends and family members about carbohydrates being "good" or "bad." This chapter will help you evaluate **what is right for you and your health.**

CHAPTER ONE

THE IMPORTANCE OF BLOOD-SUGAR AND INSULIN REGULATION

I t used to be the common wisdom that only people with diabetes or who were considered at risk for diabetes needed to be concerned with blood-sugar regulation. Now we know that keeping blood sugar well regulated is important to everyone's health, whether diabetes is indicated or not.

The disease of diabetes is actually just one point, one set of symptoms on a continuum of declining health. But the same diet, the same imbalance in your body that can cause diabetes is also strongly linked with many other symptoms of poor health. In my clinical practice, people who follow diets that keep their blood sugar well-regulated experience improvements in weight, diabetes, hypertension, cholesterol levels, depression, chronic fatigue, fibromyalgia, joint aches and pains, gastric reflux, headaches, ADD and ADHD, thyroid conditions, and many other conditions. The doctors of many of my clients have eliminated or reduced medication prescribed for these conditions because the diet that focuses on blood sugar regulation is so successful at treating the underlying cause of the problems. Even people address practical challenges, such as travelling, stocking your refrigerator, freezer, and pantry, and getting organized to make healthy cooking efficient and healthy eating convenient. These chapters are written for people who cook—and those who don't. Chapter Nine is for those who are ready to step up their healthy cooking. Here you'll find menu ideas, step-by-step plans for doing a week's worth of cooking at once without impaling yourself on a knife, and suggestions for creatively turning the same food into different dishes. Chapter Ten will tell you how to satisfy your taste for something sweet.

All of the recipes more complicated than a hard-boiled egg are included in the COOKBOOK section. For those who have rarely visited their kitchen I have included the most basic of instructions. Even if you have cooked, many people are unfamiliar with cooking methods and techniques for working with whole, fresh foods—leafy greens like kale or collards, nuts and seeds, healthy fats such as flaxseed oil, natural sweeteners like the herb stevia. The Cookbook and the GLOSSARY will provide information on what these foods are, where you can find them, and how you can prepare them.

The first appendix discusses the topic of supplements and herbs. The second appendix contains a compilation of any website or book resource mentioned within the book as well as some additional good references.

Use this book as you would your refrigerator or pantry. It will hold the information you need and you can come here whenever your appetite for change surfaces. Sometimes you might just want a snack, other times a meal. One day you may eat a lot, the next day very little. Always allow yourself time to digest; it's never wise to eat on a full stomach!

that would nourish us and keep us healthy with much less disease, depression, obesity, emotional problems, and reliance on medications.

The NUTRITION MAGIC sections are designed to help you take the information from Understanding Your Body and apply it to your diet. In Nutrition Magic you will find very specific food information, such as good sources of protein, how to incorporate healthy fats into your diet, or which foods can trigger depression. This section is also your step-by-step guide for making dietary changes. Every time you see an apple symbol, it will be followed either by a recommendation to make a small change in your diet or perform a task to support the changes you want to make (such as doing a "kitchen cupboard makeover.") The changes marked by the apple symbol are ordered in the way that I have found to be the easiest and most immediately rewarding for people. There is no timeline for making these changes other than your own. It may take you three days or three weeks to implement a step; you're not "good or bad" for doing it faster or slower. Each step will make you feel better and it's your choice to balance that goal against whatever discomfort or inconvenience you feel from making any given change.

It has always been my philosophy that changing one's diet should be a process of adding in, rather than taking away, whenever possible. This both eliminates a sense of deprivation and anxiety and provides nourishment to balance the body. When the body becomes more balanced, the desire for foods that deplete rather than nourish fades away and a lot of the struggle of changing one's diet is removed.

The MOVING FORWARD sections found in the first seven chapters focus on the nonfood aspects of change that relate to or support changing your diet and your health. For example, the first two Moving Forward sections discuss how we incorporate or get rid of beliefs and attitudes that either support or sabotage change. Other chapters take a look at sleep and overcoming sleep difficulties and exercising effectively to increase fat burning or to improve cardiovascular health. The walking puzzle-piece symbols indicate a structured task that you can work on, such as replacing your inner critic with an inner cheerleader, figuring out your target heart rate and ideal target exercise zones, or planning a strategy to improve your sleep. Unlike in the Nutrition Magic sections, the order in which you try the Moving Forward exercises is less critical. See what resonates with you and choose your own order.

The rest of the book is exclusively devoted to helping you get accustomed to a new way of eating and gradually expanding your comfort with and proficiency at feeding yourself well. Chapters Seven and Eight

REFINED CARBOHYDRATES, THE PREDIGESTED FOOD

Carbohydrates are broken down beginning in your mouth and continuing as the food passes through your digestive tract. This food group, when converted through digestion, provides glucose (blood sugar) for your body to use in a variety of ways. How much glucose is provided and how quickly depends on the type and quantity of carbohydrate you have eaten.

The bulk of daily calories for many people comes from refined carbohydrates, or what I call "predigested foods." Refined carbohydrates are foods in the carbohydrate category that have undergone any number of processes in their manufacturing to make them into a "convenience food" or to change some of their essential characteristics to make them more marketable. Bread and bread products are refined because the original kernel of whole grain has been stripped of many of its outer layers then ground up into a fine powder and often bleached white to make it more appealing to the consumer. Potato chips are refined because the original potato has been thinly sliced then fried in oil. Sugar is perhaps the ultimate refined carbohydrate. Sugar cane is processed to produce cane juice, which is then dehydrated, crystallized, and bleached into a very concentrated substance.

I call refined foods "predigested" because, in their manufacturing, the pulverizing, heating, pressing, bleaching, or stripping away of ingredients has left very little work for the body to do. Once that cereal, bagel, pasta, or corn chip hits your mouth and mixes with saliva, it's well on its way to being broken down into glucose, the eventual fate of all carbohydrate foods. The problem with refined carbohydrates is they supply your body with a lot of glucose, all at once. There are also some nonmanufactured carbohydrates (such as white potatoes) which by their very nature turn quickly into glucose. But your body is designed to receive glucose slowly, in small amounts, as the food you eat progresses through your digestive system. What may be a convenience food to you in terms of time is in actuality a serious inconvenience to you in terms of your health.

IDENTIFYING REFINED OR PREDIGESTED CARBOHYDRATES

- Flour-based products, such as pasta, bread, cookies, crackers, muffins, cakes and other baked goods, biscuits, pancakes, hamburger buns, and bagels
- Sugar-containing products, such as candy, soda pop, ice cream, frozen yogurt
- Grain products that have been pulverized, ground, or stripped, such as cold cereals, white rice, instant oatmeal, quick-cooking cereals, corn meal
- White potatoes
- Many frozen entrees (including "diet" types) containing pasta, rice, or potatoes, pizzas, snack foods
- Snack foods, such as pretzels, popcorn, corn chips, cheese curls, veggie chips, oven-baked chips, rice cakes

---

CARBOHYDRATES: ENERGY, BACK-UP FUEL, OR FAT

Your body needs glucose and uses it in any of three ways, but there is a specific order to how the glucose gets used up. How much glucose your body can use is unique to you and depends on your state of health, your size, and your physical and mental activity level. Since usage is based on these very individual factors, the idea of a fixed percentage of carbohydrates in your diet is not useful, because that particular amount of carbohydrate may not meet *your* specific needs. This is true whether we are talking about the food pyramid, the Atkins Diet, or anything in between.

For glucose to be utilized, it needs an assistant, and that assistant is the hormone insulin, which is produced by the pancreas. Insulin gets released into your bloodstream whenever your blood-glucose level rises, which means whenever you eat carbohydrate-containing foods. The amount of insulin released depends on the amount of glucose in your blood. Insulin assists the glucose in getting into your cells. It does this by making your cells more receptive to glucose passing through their walls.

THE THREE USES FOR GLUCOSE IN THE ORDER THEY OCCUR ARE:

1) to supply **energy** your cells can use immediately

2) to supply **back-up fuel** stored in your muscles and your liver, called **glycogen**

3) to supply **body fat**, for when food is needed but unavailable

---

Glucose gets supplied to your cells for energy, as your blood, enriched from the food you've recently eaten, passes through your body, including your brain. Your cells, with the help of insulin, take in glucose to fuel all the body's activities. This includes all of the ongoing functions your body does without your help, such as breathing, digesting, cell division and repair, hormone creation, etc. It also includes more conscious activities, like physical movement and thinking. Your brain is using up glucose right now as you read and make sense of this information. And I hope, as you read, you're breathing, using a little more glucose!

Glycogen, the second "stop off" point of blood-glucose, is the back-up fuel your body will be able to convert back to glucose if your blood sugar gets low. Blood sugar gets low for lots of reasons; some are healthy and normal, like the fact that you sleep for six or eight hours with no food intake, or that you exercised, using up extra amounts of fuel. It can also drop for unhealthy reasons, which we'll go into shortly. Glycogen stored in your muscles turns into glucose and supplies energy to the muscles. Liver glycogen turns into and supplies glucose to the bloodstream for all nonmuscular body functions, including those of the brain.

How much glycogen you can store will depend on two factors—how big your "storage tanks" are and how empty or full they are when you eat carbohydrates. You can't do much about the storage capacity of your liver; that pretty much stays the same. But the glycogen storage capacity of your muscle goes up the more muscle mass you develop and down as you lose muscle mass. If you're making the connection that the more muscle you have, the more your body can use carbohydrates, you're on the right track! But there's more. Glycogen gets used during heavy exercise, such as strength training, endurance activities, like long-distance running and bicycling for extended periods, or activities that consist primarily of quick bursts of movement, such as soccer, basketball, gymnastics, or ice hockey. If you don't regularly engage in one or more activities of this type, your glycogen stores don't get used very much, meaning that not much additional glucose can be stored in your muscles. So activity level is a critical factor in how well your body can use up the carbohydrates you eat.

The last place glucose can go is into your fat cells. Fat cells are designed to hold fuel for long-term storage, so that they can supply us with that fuel during times of fasting or famine. Unfortunately, many people whose diets supply too much glucose for their health, size, and activity level are steadily increasing their supply of fat. Is this happening to you?

INSULIN AND FAT STORAGE

Insulin, as you just learned, makes a great escort for glucose to enter and expand your fat cells. As long as you supply your body with more glucose than it can burn off in the hours after you eat it, it's destined to become fat. Not a pretty thought, is it? But wait, there's more you need to know.

Insulin is known as a *storage hormone*. This means it helps your body store fat. The important thing to understand here is if your food gives more glucose than you can use in the hours after eating, that extra glucose will turn to fat. And, the insulin, with its fat-storing tendencies, makes your fat cells quite possessive of their contents. In fact, even if you exercise, you won't start burning fat until your insulin level drops.

If you do exercise, have you noticed it doesn't seem to be making quite the dent in your body fat you thought it would? And perhaps you've noticed the "official" recommendations for exercise keep increasing in number of times per week and duration. A big reason for this is many people cannot tap into their fat stores because their diets, high in refined carbohydrates, produce lots of glucose, which in turn triggers lots of insulin to be released. Fortunately, exercise is one of the things that will help insulin levels drop, but this need to get rid of excess insulin prolongs the time one must exercise before moving into the fat-burning zone.

HYPOGLYCEMIA

Hypoglycemia is just a fancy word for low blood sugar. You may be familiar with what low blood sugar feels like. Ever want to put your head down on your desk for a snooze around 10 AM or 3 PM? Do you find yourself looking for a little "pick-me-up" in the form of something sweet or caffeinated? Maybe you find there are times of the day when:

- your thinking isn't as clear as it could be
- you frequently get a headache
- you're more indecisive
- the kids or a request from a coworker can easily fray your last nerve
- you want to crawl inside your refrigerator and inhale when you arrive home from work
- you're exhausted
- you crave sugar or carbohydrates

- CAROLYN complained that every day for the past four years she had a headache by 11 AM
- At work, VICKI found herself craving a candy bar about 3 PM every day.
- NANCY couldn't understand why she binged as soon as she got home from work.

RECOGNIZE ANYONE YOU KNOW? You don't have to wait for a doctor to tell you that you have hypoglycemia. If you frequently experience some of the symptoms above, it's very likely you are suffering from low blood sugar related to your diet.

Hypoglycemia occurs when the body experiences a big increase in blood-glucose and the pancreas secretes an equally large amount of insulin to deal with it. The body regards a high blood-glucose level as a state of imbalance, one that it regards as an emergency. So it reacts strongly to bring the body back into balance by clearing all the glucose out of the bloodstream. A surge of insulin causes blood-glucose to fall rapidly and sharply, and in that valley, one experiences the symptoms of hypoglycemia.

Unfortunately, what most people do when they experience low blood sugar is to look for something easy and available to pick them up. Usually, this ends up being some type of refined carbohydrate that sends blood-glucose levels right up again and begins the cycle anew. Drops in blood sugar lead a person to feel hungry and looking for food frequently throughout the day. They also can have a profound effect on mood, concentration, energy level, and the ability to respond to stress.

ASK YOURSELF THESE QUESTIONS:

1. Do I regularly eat bread, bagels, pasta, baked goods, snack foods, candy, or fat-free items such as rice cakes, puffed cereals, and frozen yogurt? __Yes __No

2. Do I drink soda or diet soda pop, fruit juices, or coffee/tea with sugar or artificial sweeteners added? __Yes __No

3. Have I been putting on weight over time that I seem unable to lose? __Yes __No

4. Despite exercising and following seemingly healthy eating habits, am I having trouble losing extra body fat? __Yes __ No

5. Do I experience the symptoms of hypoglycemia—fatigue, indecisiveness, irritability, headaches, lack of clarity in thinking, ravenous hunger, cravings for sweets and carbohydrates, mood swings, frequent eating, late-afternoon or evening bingeing? __Yes __No

If you've answered yes to any of these questions, chances are your body chemistry is out of balance due to your diet. Without attention and adjustment, you may be on your way to more serious health consequences, potential problems that are entirely avoidable with some changes to your nutritional lifestyle.

CELLULAR REBELLION: INSULIN RESISTANCE AND HYPERINSULINEMIA

Our bodies are truly amazing. They can withstand the abuse of junk food, erratic eating patterns, lack of exercise, inadequate sleep for long periods of time, and, like a trusty steed, carry us through life with barely a falter. But even though it may appear that everything is business as usual, a body's supply of health slowly erodes if daily habits deplete more than they replenish. Eventually, cells that are subjected to a daily onslaught of glucose and insulin, to highs and lows in blood sugar, fight back.

Want to know what happens when your cells rebel? Your cells are like the citizens of any country. When they're feeling oppressed, they're likely to form a resistance movement. In the case of your body, it's called *insulin resistance.*

Tired of being subjected to years of insulin overload, exhausted from being driven to remove more and more glucose from the bloodstream, your cells become less and less responsive to insulin. If this happens, your blood-sugar levels remain too high for too long after you eat a high carbohydrate meal or snack, which triggers the pancreas to secrete even more insulin. This excess insulin, dispatched in response to eating carbohydrates, is called *hyperinsulinemia.* Richard and Rachel Heller, medical doctors who wrote *The Carbohydrate Addict's LifeSpan Program* as well as several other well-known titles, state that in their research they found 75 percent of all overweight people and 40 percent of normal weight people to have insulin resistance and hyperinsulinemia.

The line between hyperinsulinemia and Type II, or so-called adult-onset diabetes, is thin. In fact, many doctors now recognize that hyperinsulinemia is "prediabetes." Eventually, a hyperinsulinemic person who doesn't change his or her diet will need medication to help the body deal with glucose. And if a cell rebellion doesn't get the person's attention, if his or her diet continues to overstress the body's insulin-producing pancreas, it too may join the revolution and eventually just quit producing insulin. Once the insulin-producing cells of the pancreas give out, the only choice left is to use insulin from an outside source. This is known as insulin-dependent diabetes.

A diet that controls blood sugar and insulin can reverse the progression of both noninsulin- and insulin-dependent diabetes. (While it cannot cause someone who is insulin dependent to no longer need insulin, diet can lower the amount of insulin needed.) One of the scariest and saddest parts of diabetes is the progressive deterioration that can happen in vision, circulation, and kidney function and the increased risk of stroke and heart disease. These complications can be avoided in most cases if blood-sugar levels are kept from elevating out of a normal range.

But diabetes is far from the only illness linked to a diet that produces too much glucose and insulin.

HYPERINSULINEMIA AND HEART DISEASE

Hyperinsulinemia is one of the most significant risks of cardiovascular disease according to the American Heart Association, which released a statement to that effect in 2000. Up until now, *fat* has been considered the number one culinary culprit. But research, and the clinical experience of a growing number of doctors and nutritionists, are showing that controlling blood sugar and insulin levels can significantly lower cholesterol levels, blood pressure, and levels of body fat. It's also becoming more evident that the most harmful effects of fat are linked to a diet high in refined carbohydrates that elevates glucose levels beyond what the body can effectively use in the hours after eating.

In many people, well-regulated blood-sugar levels can improve or eliminate symptoms of fatigue, depression, anxiety, attention deficit disorder, gastric reflux (heartburn), premenstrual syndrome, menopause, hypothyroid, fibromyalgia, mood swings, depression, headaches, irritable bowel syndrome, and joint aches and pains. Researchers may not understand yet all the mechanisms involved in making this so, but the connection is most certainly there.

Do you have any of these health problems? Are you taking or have you been told you need to take medication for any of these conditions? While medication can relieve many symptoms of a degenerative health condition, it usually doesn't address the underlying imbalance in your body or your lifestyle that is producing the symptoms. So while your symptoms may disappear, behind the scenes, your body is still struggling with the imbalance and the declining health that results.

Sandy, a seventy-one-year-old client of mine with a determination to improve her health, was on many medications for blood pressure, cholesterol and Type II diabetes. She came to me hoping to stop the progression of her diabetes symptoms, which included blood-sugar levels in the high 200's—double the normal blood-sugar range of 80-100. She was particularly concerned about tingling and occasional numbness in her feet. She had already had two heart attacks and knew her diabetes and uncontrolled blood sugar increased her risk for another.

In our initial appointment, we discussed which foods cause blood-sugar levels to increase, and I recommended she avoid these foods and increase her intake of protein. After one month of following these suggestions, her blood-sugar levels were consistently between the 120's and 140's, even occasionally dipping below 120. We tweaked her diet a bit more at our follow-up session at six weeks. Two weeks later she called to tell me that her blood-sugar levels were consistently between 80 and 100, and her doctor had taken her off one of her two diabetes medications. We expect she'll be coming off the second one soon.

Carla came to see me because, after years of living with more than a hundred extra pounds, an underfunctioning thyroid, high cholesterol, high blood pressure, depression, joint aches and pains, and gastric reflux, she was ready to take action. By her own admission, she felt skeptical about another "diet." At age forty-nine, she knew dieting didn't work and only made things worse for her. After understanding the role of blood-sugar regulation in affecting her health, she tentatively committed to giving my suggestions a try.

In less than a week she noticed her mood was better and she had a lot more energy. For the first time in years, she had energy left over at the end of the workday, instead of coming home and dropping from exhaustion. She was able to use this energy to begin a walking program, as well as to tend to other areas of her life that needed attention. Within three weeks all noticeable symptoms of her reflux were gone, and shortly thereafter her doctor agreed she no longer needed medication. At her physical, about three months into her new nutritional lifestyle, her blood pressure had dropped, she had lost 28 pounds, and her cholesterol and blood lipid numbers had improved.

Eighteen months later, she had lost sixty pounds and had great blood lipid numbers, and her doctor cut back her thyroid medication twice because her thyroid was working more on its own. She now has an active exercise program, including strength training and playing one-on-one basketball with her husband. Even in periods when the scale shows no loss of pounds, her body continues to burn fat and look more toned. Probably as significant as the health changes is the fact that she doesn't feel like she is dieting and feels confident that her eating style is one she can live with and enjoy.

You'll learn more about the nutritional changes these women made in the next section and throughout this book.

AGING OR NUTRITION DEFICIT?

Medication or surgery may have been presented to you as the treatment for your health problems. Or you may have been told your problems are "just a part of aging." But your body is not suffering from a medicine deficit; in most cases it *is* suffering from a long-standing nutrition deficit. In some cases, if enough damage has been done, medication or surgery will be necessary. In other cases medication may be helpful in the short term to protect you until the imbalances can be corrected through diet and exercise. But in most cases, a lifetime of medication and their side effects is not necessary if you are willing to choose foods that support rather than deteriorate your health.

If there were lifestyle changes you could make that would restore balance and health to your body, would you make them? The Nutrition Magic section will show you what those lifestyle changes are and help you start putting them into practice in your life. The Moving Forward section will help you look at your willingness and readiness to make changes.

NUTRITION MAGIC

"It only takes one person to change your life—you."
-Ruth Casey

Before we get going on concrete nutritional changes, I want to encourage you to make changes that will lead you to feel better. Just remember you, and only you, can find the pace that works for you. In my practice, I have found that people typically need two or three weeks to get going and get comfortable with the changes suggested in each Nutrition Magic section. Some take more time, some less. Your pace will depend on how much energy you choose to focus on making changes, as well as how big a leap the suggested change is from where you are right now. Generally, the more depleted your health, the more impact small changes will have.

> Each step you take plants a seed for change. As more and more seeds get planted, your garden of health becomes fuller. Every plant you tend is an important part of your garden. No one plant alone makes the whole.

 FOOD LOGS

Letting yourself know and honestly see what it is you're doing with food can be difficult, but if you are serious about changing, it is an important first step. I know you know how easy it is to be unconscious about food. It's also possible to be very aware of what you're eating but not aware of ways that it may be affecting your health. Recording what you eat keeps your intention to improve your diet and your health front and center in your consciousness. The details of your records will allow you to make connections between what you eat and how you feel. It will also allow you to identify any food that may be causing you problems (such as mood swings, gastric problems, sinus congestion, headaches, etc.) or a food that triggers cravings for overeating or eating foods that aren't healthy.

Copy and use the blank food log sheet on page 14 to record what you eat and drink every day. Include the time you ate and the approximate amounts. In the observation column, jot down any body observations or sensations you have. This could include things such as energy level, moods, aches and pains, changes in symptoms of any condition you have, reactions to food, etc. Also, in the activity box, record any physical activity you do, whether it's "exercise," work-related tasks, housework, walking the dog, etc.

Whether you choose to maintain food logs over the long term is up to you. People who make this level of commitment generally have more success.

DAILY FOOD LOG   DATE _____

Time	Amount & Food or Beverage	Observations:

Activities:

I suggest that you try this for at least one month. It can also be a tool you use periodically to help yourself stay or get back on track.

GLYCEMIC INDEX AWARENESS

In the last section, I talked a lot about the importance of blood-sugar regulation. But how does the average person accomplish this? Without drawing blood every time you eat to analyze its glucose level, how can you easily keep a handle on this? By becoming familiar with which carbohydrates cause large rises in blood sugar and insulin, and which ones cause moderate or small reactions, any person can make choices that will maintain healthy blood-sugar levels for them.

The *glycemic index (GI)* is an objective measure of how steeply and how quickly a given carbohydrate elevates your blood-sugar level in comparison to white bread or white sugar. To create the GI, scientists originally gave test subjects a certain amount of glucose, then observed how much their blood sugar levels rose in response. This level of blood sugar elevation was assigned a value of 100. Later, white bread was used instead of sugar, but white bread caused a blood sugar elevation that was only 70 percent of that caused by glucose, or sugar. Despite this difference, white bread was also given a value of 100.

A few hundred carbohydrate-containing foods have been tested and assigned a glycemic index number relative to either white bread or white sugar. The GI number of each food tested indicates what percentage rise in blood sugar (relative to white bread or white sugar) occurs when the specific food is eaten. Foods that have as much or more impact on blood sugar as white bread or white sugar do are in the high-glycemic category. Most manufactured or refined foods are in this category. Whole grains, fruit, and root vegetables, such as carrots, beets, and potatoes are typically moderately glycemic, with the exception of parsnips, which are high glycemic. Most other vegetables and most beans are low glycemic.

You may have deduced that knowing actual GI numbers is not a very useful tool in menu planning, since there can be a lot of variability depending on whether white bread or white sugar was used as the standard. It's also very cumbersome to learn or look up the GI rating of every food you want to eat. But identifying food generally as high, moderate, or low glycemic is very helpful for the individual person who wants to choose foods that are appropriate for him or her.

A tool that I developed for my clients to simplify things is the *Carbohydrate Chart* on page 17. The foods on this chart are listed in descending order as to their impact on blood-sugar level. You will see that almost all the foods on the upper half of the page are manufactured foods. Notice the box on the lower half of the page. The foods within this box are moderate- and low-glycemic foods, meaning they will keep blood sugar stable and insulin levels low.

It is still important to limit the amounts of food in the upper five rows within the box; how much you limit them will depend on individual factors and your health goals. You will learn in later chapters how to hone in what your body needs. For now your task is simply to become more accustomed to thinking about carbohydrates in terms of their effect on your blood.

BECOMING CARBOHYDRATE CONSCIOUS

Use the Carbohydrate Chart on page 17 to become more aware of how much carbohydrate you eat during the day and where it falls in relationship to "the box." This increases your attention to the blood sugar-raising quality of carbohydrates and helps you become more aware of the choices you make. This in turn will help prepare you for making different choices over the next several weeks. You do not need to immediately change anything you are doing now if you don't feel ready. My experience with my clients is that the simple process of becoming more aware gently leads you to gradual changes.

THE POWER OF PROTEIN

When I consult with a client I ask to see a three-day food log. In just about every case, I find the person is not eating enough protein. And, almost always, this person is having trouble with their moods, energy level, weight, or all three. Eating small amounts of protein (2 to 4 ounces) periodically

CARBOHYDRATE CHART

SUGARS

White	Confectioner's	Dextrin	Rice Syrup
Fructose	Cane Juice	Raisin Juice	Barley Malt
Dextrose	Sucanat	Sucrose	Lactose
Maltose	Fruit Juice Concentrate	Mannitol	Glucose
Turbinado	Malto-Dextrin	Beet Sugar	Sorbitol
Xylitol	Maple Syrup	Brown Sugar	Date Sugar
Molasses	Fructo-oligosaccharides	Raw Sugar	Corn Syrup

Also: Candy, Soda Pop, Fruit Juice, Fat-Free Frozen Yogurt and Sorbet, Dairyless Ice Cream

DRIED FRUIT
Banana, Mango, Apricot, Raisin, Date, Fig, Cherry, etc.

CEREALS
Flaked, Puffed, Hot Cooked (e.g., cream of wheat, cream of rice), Granola

CRACKERS & SNACK FOODS
Pretzels, Corn Chips, Veggie Chips, Popcorn, Cheese Curls, Potato Chips, Rice Cakes
(Fat-Free versions of snack foods are higher glycemic than those with fat.)

ALL REFINED FLOUR PRODUCTS
All Baked Goods including Cookies, Cakes, Muffins, Breads, Bagels, Pasta

WHOLE GRAINS
Wild Rice, Brown Rice, Oats, Quinoa, Buckwheat, Barley, Bulghur, Cous-Cous

BEANS & LEGUMES
Lentils, Kidney, Garbanzo, Black, Split Peas, White, Lima, Pinto, Navy

DENSE, STARCHY VEGETABLES
Pumpkin, Winter Squash, Sweet Potato, Yam, Peas, Corn, White Potato

FRUIT
Berries, Pears, Apples, Stone Fruits, Kiwi, Citrus, Melons, Banana, Pineapple

ROOT VEGETABLES
Carrot, Rutabaga, Celery Root, Jerusalem Artichoke, Beet, Turnip, Burdock, Parsnip

ABOVE-GROUND COMPACT VEGETABLES
Cabbage, Broccoli, Cauliflower, Brussel Sprouts, Artichoke,

ABOVE-GROUND WATERY VEGETABLES
Lettuce, Tomato, Cucumber, Kale, Collards, Mustard Greens, Swiss Chard, Bok Choy, Mushrooms, Chinese Cabbage, Radishes, Asparagus, Summer Squash, Spaghetti Squash, Eggplant, Celery, Peppers

OTHER FACTORS THAT AFFECT BLOOD SUGAR

- Fiber has no effect on blood sugar or insulin, so foods with a lot of fiber are a great choice (vegetables are typically high fiber)
- Foods that are less dense with a higher water content have little effect on blood sugar (again, think vegetables, especially those types that grow above the ground)
- Foods with less water and more sugar, natural or otherwise, have more of an impact on blood sugar (underground root vegetables, starchy root and above-ground vegetables, processed, sweetened foods, e.g., cereals, baked goods)
- Cooking or dehydrating a food concentrates its natural sugars, making it higher glycemic than the same food in its raw state (raisins/grapes, cooked carrots/raw carrots, vegetable soup/salad, tomato sauce or paste/ tomatoes)

throughout the day can do a lot to maintain consistent energy and focus. Americans have gotten away from eating protein in large part, I believe, due to unfounded but widely promoted fears about fat (more on this in the next chapter). But other reasons play a part as well, such as the need for quick and nonperishable foods that can be eaten on the run, less interest in or time for cooking, and the erroneous belief that protein damages kidneys.

Protein is absolutely essential for feeling your best and maintaining optimal health. The amino acids that make up protein are used by the body to make muscle, build and repair tissue, and create all the brain chemicals that affect mood, concentration, memory, and more. The addition of protein to meals and snacks helps keep blood sugar more stable. Lack of adequate protein is one of the most common dietary mistakes I see and is connected to one of the chief complaints of today—fatigue. It bears mentioning that the fat in protein is not an evil substance waiting to sabotage your health. To the contrary, it has some critical health functions as you will see in Chapter Two, "Fat Fiction, Lean Fact."

There is no question that to include perishable food, such as meat, fish, eggs, or cheese in your diet, you will have to give a little thought and planning to what you eat. But as you will see throughout this book, making it healthy and making it convenient and quick do not have to be incompatible.

And you will find that the benefits of eating protein regularly throughout your day will make it well worth the small amount of extra effort it takes.

DOES PROTEIN CAUSE KIDNEY DAMAGE?

This myth has been floating around for decades. It is derived from research done on people with already damaged kidneys. If you have kidneys that are not healthy, you must watch your protein intake, and your physician or a nutritionist should advise you about doing this. However, there is no evidence that protein in any amount causes damage to healthy kidneys. There is, however, evidence that high blood sugar can lead to kidney damage, which is why kidney disease is often a complication of diabetes.

ADDING PROTEIN

Protein boosts energy and concentration and supports neurochemical formation, tissue repair, and muscle growth. Eating more protein is typically the easiest change for people to make, one that quickly results in feeling better. Most people I work with remark how surprised they are at how much more energy they begin to have in a matter of days.

Start focusing on eating lean protein at each meal and, if desired, at snacks. Try to have 3 to 5 ounces at each meal, 1 to 2 ounces for snacks. Quantities of food, of course, are different for each person depending on variables of weight, activity, and individual health, but these are reasonable starting points for most people. See the list below for good sources of protein as well as some other notes and guidelines related to healthy sources of protein.

CONCERNS ABOUT MEAT AND E. COLI

There has been much concern in recent years about the presence of E. coli in meat and its potential to infect humans. E. coli is a bacteria which is usually present in the intestinal tract of both animals and humans. However, it is present in significantly higher amounts in grain-fed than in grass-fed cattle. Grain feeding creates a more acidic environment in the intestines. An acid intestinal environment would normally kill E. coli, but because of grain feeding, the bacteria become used to it and therefore resistant. This is similar

HEALTHY PROTEIN SOURCES

Lean Red Meat	Egg White
Turkey	Whey Protein Powder
Chicken	Egg White Protein Powder
Ostrich	Lamb
Buffalo, Beefalo	Lean Pork and Ham
Canned Tuna	Low-Fat Cheese
Canned Salmon	Full-Fat Cheese (less frequently)
Eggs	Cottage Cheese and Ricotta Cheese

Fresh Fish, especially cold-water types such as mackerel, herring, salmon, tuna, anchovies, sea bass and sardines

1. Try to avoid meat, fish, and poultry that have preservatives, such as sodium nitrite and nitrate, MSG, BHT, etc.
2. Bacon, ham, and deli meats are often cured with sugars. Look for plain- or herb-roasted varieties instead.
3. Animals that have been grazed, rather than farm-factory raised (grain-fed), have significantly less saturated fat, significantly more healthy essential fatty acids, and much less chance of carrying E. coli or other pathogens.
4. Nuts and nut butters have protein, but think of them as fat since that is the predominant type of calorie in them.
5. Cheese should be viewed as a higher-fat protein.
6. Many people find dairy foods aggravate allergies, asthma, PMS, menopausal difficulties, arthritis, and other conditions. Dairy can quickly add a fair amount of saturated fat to the diet, so should be used mindfully. Also, nonorganic dairy (as well as meat, poultry, and eggs) contain hormones and pesticides.
7. Tofu and other soy foods contain substances called trypsin inhibitors, which interfere with protein digestion. They also contain a lot of phytoestrogens, which in large quantities can disrupt thyroid and endocrine function. This is more likely to happen as people eat more soy-fortified foods. Many people find soy foods cause gas and bloating. They're best used sparingly.
8. Eat fish several times a week for its rich DHA (essential fatty acid) content.
9. The dark meat on poultry, while higher in fat, contains a lot of zinc which your brain needs.
10. Keep in mind that saturated fat is not evil. When the body is not loaded with glucose and insulin, your body is much better able to process fat.

to the way certain strains of bacteria have become resistant to antibiotics due to their overuse.

Most commercially raised cattle are fed grain to fatten the animal. Organic or free-range cattle are allowed to graze and eat on pasture grass. Grazing not only results in cows that have less resistant E. coli, but it also produces meat with less saturated fat and more of the desirable healthy fats. Visit the website **www.eatwild.com** to learn more about the health benefits of pasture-based farming.

The condition of your immune system plays a big part in whether E. coli will actually make you sick or not. You are exposed to pathogens of many types, every day. Whether or not you get sick depends on your level of health and your body's ability to resist infection, both of which are enhanced with good nutrition.

MOVING FORWARD

PREPARING YOURSELF FOR CHANGE

The process of changing how you eat is a much bigger undertaking than is usually presented in books, magazines, and by most health professionals. Most people fail at making significant long-term changes because so little attention and support is given to the process of change. Instead, people are handed a "diet" and expected to go home and follow it. In reality, big behavioral changes rarely happen in a linear progression. Most people don't just decide to change one day, then proceed without any bumps and backsliding. But I know I don't need to tell you that!

How and what you eat is intricately woven into your past, your social relationships, work setting and patterns, emotions, finances, cooking knowledge and interest, and family demands. To be successful at change, you have to be willing to patiently work on each piece of the puzzle as it presents itself. Sometimes you can work on a few pieces at a time; sometimes you only have attention for one. But to expect yourself to do it all at once is unrealistic; then to blame yourself for failing is simply unkind.

The idea that you are either "on" or "off" your diet is part of the dieting mentality that has been so damaging to so many. You will have days you are able to make better choices, days you make less healthy ones. Sometimes a "bad" day will have to do with external circumstances, but in most cases a bad day is related to one of two things:

1. Not thinking and planning ahead to take care of your food needs
2. Emotional eating

This program can help you with each one of these, but you have to supply the patience and commitment to keep moving forward.

PLANNING TO BE SUCCESSFUL

Change is made up of small steps that add up over time. The *success assessment* is a tool to help you think more consciously about all the individual little steps that go into making a larger, nutritional lifestyle change.

SUCCESS ASSESSMENT

Go through the success assessment on the following pages and identify the steps you will need to make in the coming weeks and months. These steps can then form your weekly goals.

This self-assessment is designed to help you think about changes necessary to reach your desired goals of good health. This tool encourages you to think honestly about what *you are willing to do* to improve your health. The behaviors identified in the success assessment are the ones that are exhibited by people who have long-term success at changing their diets and their health.

It is not necessary for you to make all of these changes at once; in fact, it's unlikely that you'll be successful if you try to do that. Some of these changes may take years to make; some may come easily right away. Some may be more relevant to you than others. The important thing is for you to be honest with yourself about how much effort you're willing and able to put out to get the results you want. Your answers are likely to be different depending on the circumstances of your life, so take this out periodically for a reassessment, particularly if you're not getting the results you want.

Success assessment quiz

For each item, rate yourself on a scale of 1 to 3.

1 = I'm willing and able to take this step now.

2 = I want to be able to take this step but need to do some other things first to get there

3 = I'm not willing or able to make this change.

1. Take time to seek information in one or more ways and come up with a planned approach (reading, taking classes, seeing a nutritionist, and/or committed participation in a group or program). _____
2. Make more time in my life to prepare food for myself. _____
3. Clean out my cupboards and refrigerator, identifying foods and ingredients that undermine my health. _____
4. Stock my kitchen with ingredients to make healthy meals and snacks. _____
5. Spend more money, if necessary, on fresh and whole foods that cost more than refined foods with artificial flavors and chemical preservatives. _____
6. Talk with other family members about my intention to change how I eat. _____
7. Make changes for myself even if family members are not willing to do the same for themselves. _____
8. Set a good example for my children with my food choices and teach them why it's important to eat well. _____
9. Set aside two to four hours per week (not all at once) to prepare food for rest of week. _____
10. Anticipate what my food needs are for the day ahead and make a plan to meet them as healthfully as possible. _____
11. Bring food with me when I know I'll be stuck with no access to healthy food. _____

12. Make special requests in restaurants to get a healthy meal that meets my needs. _____

13. Keep a food journal to help me make connections between what I eat and how I feel physically and emotionally. _____

14. Weigh and measure food as necessary to help visualize portion sizes. _____

15. Reduce my use of sugar and sweeteners that elevate my insulin levels.____

16. Reduce my use of refined carbohydrates, such as bread, pasta, bagels, baked goods, corn chips, etc. _____

17. Eat breakfast daily. _____

18. Expand my cooking skills. _____

19. Pay attention to my body's response to what I eat, including the use of journal writing. _____

20. Examine my emotional relationship with feeding myself. _____

21. Use nutritional supplements. _____

22. Drink water daily (1/2 ounce per pound of body weight). _____

23. Clean and organize my kitchen so it feels good to be in. ———

24. Make sure I have appropriate knives and cookware. _____

25. Create support systems in my life for making the changes I desire. _____

It may seem at first as though there are too many things you need to change. Don't be overwhelmed, but do appreciate how much effort goes into changing how you eat. The whole concept of "a diet" simply does not recognize the time and energy it takes to develop new, healthier habits. You will be more successful if you stop putting all of your focus on the food and recognize that many other parts of your life affect the food choices you make.

 WHAT ARE *YOUR* HEALTH GOALS?

Spend some time thinking about what your personal goals are for improving your health. Get very specific. Instead of saying, "I want to be healthier" or "I want to lose weight," delve into what those things mean for you. How would they affect you on daily basis?

Instead of "I want to be healthier," try "I want to be able to walk up and down the three flights of stairs at work without feeling out of breath"; or "I want to have the energy to go on a two-hour bicycle ride"; or "I want to lower my blood pressure without the use of medication." Instead of "I want to lose weight," try "I want to fit into that size-12 pair of black jeans at the bottom of my drawer" or "I want to feel comfortable wearing a tucked-in jersey."

After you have come up with some specific goals, fill in as much detail as you can. Allow yourself to imagine yourself living your goal. Fill in as much of the sensory detail as you possibly can. Create a picture in your mind's eye. Are you alone or with other people? Are people speaking to you? Is there music? Are you in a special location? What can you see around you? Do you feel anything such as breezes or sunlight on your skin? You may find that this is difficult and that you have negative messages and images getting in the way. Simply notice what those negative intrusions are—it's good information for you to have. Then let go of them. Keep trying to focus on *positive sensory detail.* Write down your goals and all the details surrounding them. Set a date that you think is reasonable for you to reach your goal and write that down too.

Successful people are those who can imagine themselves accomplishing whatever it is they want. This is a common technique athletes use to enhance their performance. Research shows that mental rehearsal of an activity in combination with actual practice is the most potent way to reach one's goals. People who are not successful do not visualize themselves being successful; instead, they allow negative thoughts and images to dominate.

Spend five minutes each day imagining yourself as you would like to be.

BELIEFS AND ATTITUDES

Many times, we hold conscious and unconscious beliefs and attitudes that keep us from being successful. When we're undertaking change, it's helpful to identify all the roadblocks that may come up. Some you will learn about as you do the goal-setting exercise above. You may already be aware of voices in your head objecting to what you imagine you may have to do to get healthier.

IDENTIFYING BARRIERS TO CHANGE

Write down all the negative messages, potential roadblocks, and challenges you feel may keep you from reaching your goals. You will work with ridding yourself of these messages in the next chapter.

CHAPTER TWO

FAT FICTION,
LEAN FACT

S ince the early sixties, we have been highly conditioned with the message "fat is bad." The viewpoint of the media, the medical journals, the pharmaceutical industry, and the food industry has been that saturated—meaning "animal"—fat causes high cholesterol. And high cholesterol, we're told, is a leading cause of heart disease.

Many scientists have long questioned the fat-heart disease hypothesis and the research used to support it, but their voices have been silenced by the chorus of "fat causes heart disease" advocates. After forty years, even those folks are acknowledging that the picture is much larger and more complex than the simple generalization that fat is bad. Fat in general, and cholesterol in particular, have some very critical functions in promoting and protecting our health, including heart health. There are many other factors beyond quantity that need to be considered in understanding how the body responds to dietary fat.

All of the "replacement fats"—the zero-cholesterol vegetable oils and margarine that we all thought were healthier—are not looking so great under the scrutiny of current research. And there is a significant amount of well-researched and published evidence demonstrating that many of the original and most often cited "cholesterol studies" do not actually support the conclusions they are reported to conclude.

One trend that has become evident is that there are also many negative health effects from too little fat and from too little of the right kinds of fat. The issue may well be not how much fat is in our diet, but what *kinds* of fat are we consuming and from what sources? Many of the fats placed on the market since the "cholesterol scare" of the last four decades we're now being told to avoid.

In "Fat Fiction, Lean Fact" we'll examine some of the current research and thinking about cholesterol, heart disease, and obesity. We'll also discuss the health impact of fat-restricting diets and the use of "replacement fats." And, of course, you'll get some guidelines for healthfully including fat in your diet in the Nutrition Magic section. The Moving Forward part of Chapter Two will give you tools to work with some of the emotional resistance of successfully changing how you eat. You will learn about how your subconscious works to both learn and unlearn negative and self-defeating thought patterns. And you will discover how you can effectively use these same techniques to supply your subconscious mind with positive, success-oriented messages.

UNDERSTANDING YOUR BODY

IT'S TIME FOR FAT-FRIENDLY THINKING

Confused about fat? Join the club. Dietary fat plays complex roles in the functioning of your brain and body, and the significance of fat to your health has been lost in the tidal wave of anti-fat messages. Accurate information about fat has been ignored or convoluted by agendas that reach far beyond the health needs of you and me. It's important to recognize that four decades of "fat is bad" thinking has produced many food products, drugs, services, and models of medical treatment that are based on the assumption that fat, particularly saturated fat, is bad for us. "Bad fat" thinking has produced a tremendous product and service economy of its own, and for that reason alone, those who challenge that way of thinking, no matter how scientifically credible, struggle to be heard. And the fact is, we simply have more information now than we've ever had about dietary fats and health, and more is continually being discovered. As frustrating as it may be that things keep changing, just remember you have a goal to be as healthy as you can be, and that means keeping up with the current knowledge.

Fats are essential to your health in so many ways. Fat is a key element in the structure of the brain, nervous system, cells, and hormones. And, surprising though this might seem, fat is necessary for your body to burn fat. Some fats, especially the saturated ones, contain antimicrobial properties that help your cells to resist infiltration by bacteria and other pathogens. Although fat is reportedly a primary cause of heart disease, studies across the globe show neither strong nor consistent evidence that a decrease in fat intake, especially animal fat intake, results in lower levels of heart disease or deaths from heart disease.

Shocked to hear this? Most people in my classes or those whom I see in my office have been religiously following low-fat diets for years or decades and find it scary, threatening, or confusing when I present this information. But most also know that what they've been doing has not been working to support their health. And it's pretty hard to ignore the fact that among U.S. women, heart disease has been steadily increasing. The number of overweight men, women, and children in the United States has been and continues to be on the rise despite the fact that fat consumption has been decreasing for forty years.

How can this be? Well, for one thing, Americans are eating significantly more refined carbohydrates than ever before. Remember the negative impact of elevated blood sugar and insulin on health we talked about in Chapter One? None of the studies on the health effects of fats ever took that factor into account. It appears that calories and fat are handled differently in your body, depending on blood sugar and insulin levels.

Second, since the "cholesterol scare" beginning in the early sixties, the grocery stores have been flooded with no-cholesterol vegetable oils, margarine to replace butter, hydrogenated and partially hydrogenated fats in a majority of foods, and enormous varieties of fat-free products. Until very recently, nobody thought to study the effects of these manufactured foods on health. Now that we are, the findings require that we rethink our whole model regarding dietary fat.

Finally, many researchers have gone back and thoroughly examined the data in many of the original studies concluding that saturated fat raises cholesterol levels and elevated cholesterol levels increase risk for heart disease. These credible scientists are critical of how the original studies were reported and strongly refute that the data support these conclusions.

So, sit back, open your mind, and prepare for an attitude adjustment about fat!

SMART, HAPPY PEOPLE EAT FAT

As a former psychotherapist, I find one of the most exciting areas in nutritional research today to be the study of the effect of food on our thoughts, emotions, and behavior. And fat plays a key role in this. Do you remember hearing when you were younger that fish is brain food? The reason is fish contains some specific types of fatty acids critical for brain functions and not found in other food sources. By "brain functions" I'm talking about several things that affect your moment-to-moment well-being, such as:

- the ability to manufacture the chemicals that regulate your moods
- the ability to process information and thoughts
- the ability to focus and concentrate
- the ability to appropriately control behavior
- the ability to direct all the physical functions of the body at the cellular level as well as the activities of organs and muscles

In addition to this, the brain itself is composed of 60 percent fat, and the source of that fat is, or should be, your diet. So what do you imagine happens to all these functions when you decide that fat is bad for you and strip most of it from your diet?

Many parts of the nervous system that carry out the brain's directives are composed of fat as well. The *myelin sheath* is the fat layer that surrounds and protects nerve fibers and helps with the transmission of nerve impulses along this information superhighway. *Nerve synapses*, the connecting link between two nerve cells, are composed of fat. When your diet contains inadequate amounts of fat or the wrong kinds of fats, all of these fat-based structures are compromised and may deteriorate, which means that all of the functions that depend on these structures suffer. There is a growing body of research linking many diseases and conditions with fatty acid deficiencies. Depression, attention deficit disorder and hyperactivity, schizophrenia, bipolar illness, diabetic neuropathy, multiple sclerosis, ALS or Lou Gehrig's Disease, stress, seizure disorders, sciatica, dementia, Alzheimer's, and many other conditions that result from diminished or impaired nerve conduction have been noted to improve with the addition of specific fats to the diet. This doesn't mean we know for a certainty that all of these conditions are caused by lack of fat or can be cured by adding it. It does mean that a fat deficiency appears to be present in each of these conditions and that symptoms frequently improve with the addition of certain types of dietary fat.

IT TAKES FAT TO BURN FAT

Fat is even necessary for your body to burn fat. Bile salts, manufactured by the liver, help break down dietary fat so your body can utilize it. Cholesterol, a type of fat I know you've heard about, is necessary for the production of bile salts.

There is another very significant way fat helps your body to burn both dietary and stored fat that researchers are more recently looking at. We actually have *two types of fat cells* in our body, white ones and brown ones. The *white fat* cells are the ones that hold gatherings around your midsection and any other places they can find to hang out, hoping someday to be needed.

Brown fat cells, however, lie deeper within your body, providing cushioning to vital organs and the spinal column. But these brown cells also have another important and very specialized function. Brown fat cells' *primary* job is to burn calories to provide heat energy for your body. That's right, these little guys and gals exist to munch on calories you take in as well as any stored fat you may have hanging around. This process of producing heat energy by burning calories is called *thermogenesis*.

Brown cells have their own metabolism, and the more revved up it is, the more efficient your body is at burning incoming food and body fat. French researchers in a 1992 study were able to measure the level of thermogenesis taking place in three groups of women: those who had no trouble with weight control, those with a history of obesity, and those who had recently experienced weight gain and were having difficulty losing the weight. What the researchers found was a clear relationship between the level of activity in the brown cells and the tendency of the body to gain and hold weight. The women with no weight problems had an increase in thermogenesis when calories were taken in (in the form of sugar water) whereas the other two groups had no increase in calorie-burning activity. The women in the group with a history of obesity not only didn't increase their brown cell metabolism, but their body stored the calories (totally unfair, I think we agree!). Well, guess what substance has been found to kick those little brown cells into working their (or your) butts off? You guessed it—fat! That's right, it takes fat to burn fat. Later we'll talk about which kind of fat accomplishes this minor miracle.

ESSENTIALLY HEALTHY

One type of fat in particular—cholesterol—is the critical component in the manufacturing of hormones. While women tend to be most aware of hormones because of reproductive cycles, hormones have a much broader impact as information chemicals that "run" the body. Insulin, discussed in Chapter One, is one example; but many more hormones are involved in reproduction, growth, metabolism, building bone density, and maintaining fluid and electrolyte balance in the body.

Did you know that nicks in your arteries are repaired with cholesterol? Cholesterol is so important that roughly 75 percent of what your body uses the liver manufactures itself, increasing or decreasing output depending on how much cholesterol you get in your diet. In fact, this is why cholesterol restriction is *not* an effective way to control blood cholesterol. Your body knows how much cholesterol you need from day to day and will override dietary attempts to manipulate its level.

Fat is also a critical component of something called *prostaglandins*, which are hormone-like regulatory substances that affect virtually every system and cell of your body. Prostaglandins are made from essential fatty acids, which are fats that we need to get from our diet because the body cannot produce enough of them on its own—that is why they're called "essential." Prostaglandins regulate things like:

- Expansion and contraction of arteries and blood vessels
- Blood thinning and clotting
- Pain transmission
- Inflammation
- Immunity
- Cell proliferation

There are two types of prostaglandins, known as "good" and "bad." These are relative terms and not exactly accurate, because we need both types; we just need them in proper balance. For example, the so-called good ones promote expansion of the arteries while the so-called bad ones cause constriction. Too many of the bad ones leading to over-contraction, and could cause what we know as a heart attack. But too much expansion would decrease pumping and circulation of blood. So we must have both types of prostaglandins to keep these opposing functions in balance.

Let's go through this list and see how the regulation of each of these functions is related to your health and could be related to various health problems.

• Expansion and contraction of arteries and blood vessels

The ability of arteries and blood vessels to expand and contract rhythmically and with flexibility is the mechanism behind pumping blood to feed every cell and function of your body. This expansion and contraction is critical to overall health and to preventing heart attacks and high blood pressure.

• Blood thinning and clotting

If blood clots too much, we run the risk of strokes; if it doesn't clot enough, wounds won't heal.

• Pain transmission and Inflammation

Pain transmission is a concern for anyone with a condition that involves chronic or temporary pain, such as fibromyalgia, arthritis, or an injury, to name a few. Allergies, arthritis, lupus, and inflammatory bowel disease all involve inflammation and are examples of conditions where the body's inability to tone down its inflammatory response is central to the symptoms of the illness.

• Immunity

In the immune system, proper regulation can make the difference between being able to fight off illness appropriately and an immune system that becomes overactive and begins to mistakenly attack itself, the central feature of autoimmune diseases like lupus, fibromyalgia, chronic fatigue.

• Cell proliferation

Wound healing, tissue repair, growth, and fetal development are examples of healthy cell proliferation. Cancer is a disease in which cell proliferation runs amuck; cancer cells grow and spread out of control.

Can you see how having enough of the proper fat in your diet to produce hormones and the right balance of prostaglandins is essential for preventing or treating many common health problems?

Still not sure it's wise to consider fat your friend? Here are a few other ways that fat supports your health. Healthy structure of your cell walls relies on having enough fat. Too little fat, especially saturated fat, theoretically the "bad boy" of all fats, causes cell membranes to become too "soft." When cell walls lack the proper amount of stiffness, they are more permeable to pathogens and carcinogens. Too much unsaturated fat, especially the polyunsaturated vegetable oils, causes cell walls to become "watery." Cell wall integrity is a vital part of keeping up your immunity to illness. And if cell walls don't provide an adequate screen against foreign invaders, then DNA, your genetic material, is more at risk for being exposed to mutating agents, including cancer.

If your body doesn't have enough fat or can't utilize it properly, your ability to use the *fat-soluble vitamins* A, E, D, and K is compromised. Among other things, each of those vitamins is important to your vision, heart health, bone structure, and blood clotting, respectively.

MOST UNFRIENDLY FATS

When cholesterol became an outlaw, there were basically two types of fats that, over the years, flooded the market: vegetable oils and hydrogenated fats. No-cholesterol oils from plants, such as canola, corn, safflower, sunflower, and the generic "vegetable" oil created a whole new industry.

Though these oils promised, in theory, more health protection than animal fats, the fact that they remained liquid made them more difficult to use in place of solid shortening, butter, or lard, particularly in baking. The industry's solution to this problem was to create hydrogenated fat, made of vegetable oils, which are chemically manipulated to become solid at room temperature. Hydrogenated fats have the "advantage" of behaving like animal fats when used in baking, which was a good thing for the manufacturers. And for commercial production of cookies, crackers, snack foods, etc., hydrogenated fats have a much longer shelf life. Actually, hydrogenated fats, such as Crisco, had been on the market for decades before; their use simply proliferated after the early cholesterol theories were advanced.

Now, thirty years after vegetable oils and hydrogenated fats were introduced into our diet, they aren't looking as healthy as once promised. In fact, in the late fifties, a researcher named Ancel Keys claimed that hydrogenated fat was the culprit in coronary heart disease. American Heart Association documents of the time also warned against consumption of hydrogenated fats. Both of these assertions triggered a public relations campaign by the edible oil industry to recreate the image of hydrogenated fat. By 1965, the American Heart Association deleted warnings about both hydrogenated fat and trans-fats from its dietary statement and Keys shifted his attention to the hypothesized relationship between saturated animal fat and heart disease. (The history of how natural saturated animal fats became evil, and manufactured fats took their place in the market, makes interesting reading, and I encourage you if you're interested to read *Know Your Fats* by Mary Enig, Ph.D. See Appendix II.)

Vegetable oil, by nature, is less stable then animal fat; vegetable oil goes rancid more easily, especially when exposed to heat, air, or light. The production of these oils typically involves temperatures over 200 degrees, pressure, which generates more heat, and exposure to light and air. Then, the resulting oil is packaged in clear glass or plastic bottles where it sits on warehouse, grocery store, and finally, your kitchen shelves. Hydrogenated oils undergo further processing. What follows is a description of how hydrogenated fats, such as margarine, are manufactured.

HYDROGENATION: This is the process that turns polyunsaturates, normally liquid at room temperature, into fats that are solid at room temperature—margarine and shortening. To produce them, manufacturers begin with the cheapest oils—soy, corn, cottonseed, or canola, already rancid from the extraction process—and mix them with tiny metal particles—usually nickel oxide. The oil, with its nickel catalyst, is then subjected to hydrogen gas in a high-pressure, high-temperature reactor. Next, soap-like emulsifiers and starch are squeezed into the mixture to give it a better consistency; the oil is yet again subjected to high temperatures when it is steam-cleaned. This removes its unpleasant odor. Margarine's natural color, an unappetizing gray, is removed by bleach. Dyes and strong flavors must then be added to make it resemble butter. Finally, the mixture is compressed and packaged in blocks or tubs and sold as a health food."

From The Skinny on Fats *by Mary Enig, Ph.D., published by the Weston A. Price Foundation, www.westonaprice.org*

Pretty unappealing isn't it, to think about putting such a food into your body? It's more than just a disgusting thought, though; the health risks and consequences of replacing naturally occurring fats with these chemical concoctions can be serious. The process of hydrogenating oils causes their molecular structure to be rearranged; we call these rearranged fats *trans-fats or trans-fatty acids.* Trans-fatty acids interfere with the body's ability to use the good, essential fatty acids. The good fatty acids are known to help lower LDL ("bad") cholesterol and raise HDL ("good") cholesterol. But the trans-fats raise LDL and lower HDL cholesterol. The greater the amount of trans-fats in the diet, the greater these effects are. The U.S. Food and Drug Administration has recognized the adverse effects of trans-fats enough to have recently ruled that, in the near future, trans-fat amounts must be included on all nutrition labeling.

It is only recently that hydrogenated or trans-fats have been called into question, so little if any research has been conducted to find out what effect they may have on the brain and nervous system. It is unlikely that our brains, as sophisticated and precise as they are, can function as well with these chemically altered fats. And what about the prostaglandins that are made from essential fatty acids? Doesn't it make sense that many of today's health problems are connected to the *lack of natural fats* in our diet?

WHAT ABOUT CHOLESTEROL?

How we currently think about the link between cholesterol and heart disease is based on two assumptions:

1) that saturated fat elevates blood cholesterol; and
2) that elevated cholesterol is linked to higher rates of heart disease

But the relationships between saturated fat and cholesterol and cholesterol and heart disease are not nearly as definitive as we have been led to believe. And even if some moderate level of relationship were to exist (which it does not), it certainly doesn't prove cause. Here are some of the facts and study results that aren't typically reported in the press, but may surprise you concerning fat, cholesterol, and health.

• According to the late pioneer heart surgeon, Michael DeBakey, one-third of patients who have coronary bypass surgery have cholesterol levels below 200.

• DeBakey also surveyed 1700 patients with hardening of the arteries (atherosclerosis) and found no relationship between blood cholesterol levels and the incidence of atherosclerosis.[1]

• Only 25 percent of the material in clogged arteries, when analyzed, is found to be saturated fat. The rest is made up of unsaturated vegetable oils.

• One of the biggest diet/heart disease studies ever conducted was the Framingham, Massachusetts, Heart Study, a long-term study involving over 6,000 people. The study, which began in 1948, has often been cited as proof of the fat-heart disease link. The director of the study, William Castelli, stated in an article reported in the *Archives of Internal Medicine*, "in Framingham, Massachusetts, the more saturated fat one ate, the more cholesterol one ate, the more calories one ate, the lower the person's serum cholesterol…the opposite of what the equations provided by Hegsted et al (1958) and Keyes et al (1957) would predict." [2]

• One of the most well-known studies, given the acronym MRFIT and sponsored by the National Heart, Lung, and Blood Institute, compared mortality rates and eating habits of over 12,000 men. A marginal reduction in coronary heart disease was shown among those who didn't smoke and followed reduced saturated fat and cholesterol diets. However, this group also showed a higher death rate overall from causes other than heart disease.[3]

---

[1] DeBakey, M, et al, *JAMA*, 1964, 189:655-59
[2] Castelli, William, *Arch Internal Medicine*, Jul 1992, 152:7: 1371-1372
[3] "Multiple Risk Factor Intervention Trial; Risk Factor Changes and Mortality
    Results," *JAMA*, Sept. 24, 1982, 248:12:1465

• A Swedish study on fat and breast cancer involving thousands of women showed no relationship between eating saturated fat and increased risk for breast cancer, but did show a strong link between use of vegetable oils and increased risk.[4]

• Extensive analysis by Harvard University Departments of Nutrition and Epidemiology of data from many of the studies that concluded saturated fats were linked with increased coronary heart disease, came up with a different picture. These researchers looked at the effect of trans-fatty acids, the type of fat found in margarine and refined, processed vegetable oils. Trans-fats had never been considered separately in these studies when they were done originally. They found that trans-fats lowered good cholesterol and raised bad cholesterol at a rate double that of saturated fat.[5]

• Several of the original studies that correlated consumption of fat with deaths from heart disease worldwide simply left out the data from countries in which the data didn't conform to the hypothesis.[6]

In addition to the many voices and studies which now contradict the demonizing of dietary fat, we can look at the nutrition and health trends for the last several decades and see that reducing the consumption of animal fat has not produced significant decreases in heart disease. Americans have been eating less fat from animal sources for the last forty years. If animal fat and cholesterol caused heart disease, we would expect to see a much tighter relationship between less fat and heart disease. But that isn't the case, in this country nor globally. Even though overall fat and animal fat consumption has decreased over the last forty years, our use of vegetable fats which are highly refined has increased dramatically. These fats appear not just in bottles, but in almost all refined, packaged products you purchase—crackers, cookies, breads, snack foods, condiments, salad dressings, margarine, microwave popcorn, "heart healthy" butter replacement spreads, and many more foods

---

[4] Wolk, et al, *Archives of Internal Medicine* 158:41
[5] Ascherio, Stampfer and Willet, *Trans-fatty Acids and Coronary Heart Disease,*
    Background and Scientific Review, Department of Nutrition, Harvard School of Public Health
[6] Ravnskov, Uffe, M.D. PhD, *The Cholesterol Myths: Exposing the Fallacy that Saturated Fat
    and Cholesterol Cause Heart Disease,* p.15-46.

that line grocery store shelves. Damaged fats, sugar, and refined carbohydrates have steadily edged out diets that contained plenty of natural fats and unprocessed, whole food.

Do you find yourself not quite willing to believe that something so ingrained in our culture's thinking could be wrong? I know that when I first began reading some of this information several years ago, I had a hard time believing it. After all, most of us have been taught to believe that a scientific or medical study is conducted with the sole purpose of finding what is "true." I would carefully check out references and look in medical journals to see if someone really had said what they had been quoted as saying. I wondered about the reputations of critics who were questioning "truths" that were so much a part of my upbringing. Like you, perhaps, I had the "fear of fat" litany so deeply ingrained that I could never have started to eat more fat without doing a lot of research on my own to convince myself I wouldn't be harming my health. Once I was reasonably convinced, I began experimenting on myself by adding more fat back into my diet, and then I introduced these new ideas and this dietary change to my clients.

I have seen only positive results, never negative. Cholesterol levels come down (although it's still unclear what "healthy" cholesterol numbers are for any given individual), weight comes off, depression lifts, thyroid function often improves, inflammatory conditions calm down, hair, skin and nails get healthier.

Of course, adding more healthy fat to the diet has to be combined with reducing sugar and refined carbohydrates, as was discussed in Chapter One. But it's time to rethink your use of fat. The Nutrition Magic section of this chapter will help you learn about how to incorporate healthy fat into your diet and guide you in eliminating health-damaging fat.

NUTRITION MAGIC

Saturated, polyunsaturated, monounsaturated, omega 3, omega 6, DHA, EPA cholesterol—all these terms for fats can get confusing and cumbersome and turn eating into a chemistry lab. There are, however, a few things I think it's important to understand so you know why you're choosing one type of fat over another.

OMEGA FATTY ACIDS

Two omega fatty acids (Omega 3, Omega 6) are also called essential fatty acids because the body cannot readily make them and we must get a substantial amount of them from dietary sources. The body can make Omega 9, a third Omega fat, so it is not labeled as essential. But Omega 9 fatty acids, like the other two, have some very essential health functions.

The Omega 3's come from cold water fish (see box, page 42) and from a few plant sources, the most abundant of which is flaxseed (sold as seed, ground meal, or oil). Omega 6 fats are abundant in nuts, seed, grains, and vegetables. Omega 9 fats make up a substantial percentage of the fats contained in avocados, olives, olive oil, peanut oil, and canola oil (only if unhydrogenated). You may also be surprised to find out that beef tallow, lard, eggs, butter, and chicken fat also contain substantial amounts of the healthy Omega 9 fats.

Here are some of the most important things for you to know about the Omega fats and your health.

1. **The Omega 3-rich fish oils** contain two subcategories of fats—EPA and DHA—that are not available anywhere else (except marine algae). It's not important that you know their names, just that you know these two fats are *critical* for healthy brain functioning. Studies and experience have shown that depression, bipolar disorder, and ADD/ADHD all improve with the addition of these fats to the diet. If you don't or won't eat fish, it is important to supplement your diet with some other source of fish oil, such as capsules.

2. **Humans need a specific ratio of Omega 6 to Omega 3 fats** in the diet in order to produce the regulatory prostaglandins we talked about in Chapter One. That ratio is four to one, or four parts of Omega 6 to one part of Omega 3. Too many Omega 6 fatty acids in the diet cause the

body to overproduce the "bad" prostaglandin type. Because Omega 6 fats are so prevalent in vegetables, the extensive use of vegetable oils— a concentrated source of Omega 6 fats—has increased the average person's ratio to something in the order of sixteen to one. Eating a varied diet including vegetables, nuts or nut butters (as in peanut butter), and some grains, as well as using olive oil, gives you ample Omega 6 fat.

3. **Almost everyone needs to make an effort to get Omega 3 fats** in order maintain the 4:1 balance. These fats are critical to so many functions of the brain and body. I can't think of anyone who wouldn't benefit from the addition of this fat to his or her diet, unless there's a medical reason he or she isn't able to metabolize fat. If you are taking blood thinning or anticoagulant medication, you should consult your health professional before taking supplements with Omega 3 oils, as they also have a blood-thinning effect. But you can still enjoy eating omega-rich fish! Most people benefit from supplementing with Omega 3 fats in the form of fish, fish oil capsules, flaxseed oil, ground flaxseeds, or some combination of these.

4. **The Omega 9 and the Omega 3 fats are cancer protective.** An excess of Omega 6 fats in the diet can make your body more vulnerable to the uncontrolled proliferation of cancer cells. Your cell membranes are also more watery and less resistant to all foreign invaders when there is too much Omega 6 fat in the diet.

FISH SOURCES OF OMEGA 3 FATTY ACIDS
(based on 3.5-ounce portions)

Best	grams	Next Best	grams	Low	grams
Salmon*	1 - 1.7	Freshwater Bass	.7	Cod	.2
Herring	1.7	Bluefish	.7	Flounder	.2
Mackerel	2.4	Carp	.6	Grouper	.2
Anchovies	1.4	Catfish	.4	Haddock	.1
Sardines	1.7	Halibut	.4	Perch	.2
Sable	1.5	Sea Bass	.6	Pike	.2
Albacore Tuna	1.5			Snapper	.3

*Farm-raised salmon can be as high as 1.9 grams, but is only a good source of Omega 3 if the fish were fed an Omega 3 rich diet.

CHOOSING FRIENDLY OVER UNFRIENDLY FATS

Most highly refined fats are not friendly to your health. This includes anything that is hydrogenated or partially hydrogenated. You will see this term on the label of margarine, some "heart healthy" spreads, salad dressings, cookies, crackers, breads, muffins, and microwave popcorn. In fact most commercially processed foods contain hydrogenated oils in them, even products carried in health food stores. That's right, margarine is not good for you—don't use it! All natural butter, in moderation, is actually good for you.

The other grouping of unhealthy fat includes most vegetable oils, such as safflower, canola, soybean, sunflower, corn, and generic vegetable oil. Why aren't these good for you? Two reasons. The first is that they provide too high a concentration of Omega 6 fats, as I discussed above. The second is that these oils are frequently damaged by their exposure to heat, light, and air in the manufacturing and packaging process. The oils become oxidized, which means their molecules are unstable. We call unstable molecules such as these *free radicals*, a term you may have heard before. Free radicals are molecules that go around your body nibbling away at edges of your cells in order to scavenge other molecules to make themselves more stable. *Free radical damage,* as this is called, makes your cells more vulnerable to being invaded by bacteria, pathogens, and carcinogens. Pesticides, pollution, stress—even good stress like exercise—causes free-radical damage to your body. Because we have so many sources of free radicals that we can't control, it's wise to minimize the ones we can. And no, I'm not suggesting you give up exercising! But there certainly are good options for oils that won't add free radicals to your body.

Another problem with oils that are made by companies not producing specifically for the organic and health food markets is that the oils are extracted from the seeds using chemical solvents.

Vegetable oils made for the health food market will be labeled "cold pressed" or "expeller pressed" and sold in opaque containers that let no light through. These oils are less likely to be damaged when you purchase them. But cold pressing and opaque containers will not solve the problem of getting too many Omega 6 fatty acids. Limiting your use of vegetable oils such as sunflower, safflower, corn, canola, or soy is the most important way you can do that.

ARE THERE GOOD OILS?

Extra virgin olive oil, sesame oil, and coconut oil are three oils that are ideal for cooking. You've probably heard that coconut oil is a very saturated fat and a definite no-no for anyone concerned with health. This is another example of painting with a broad stroke when a narrow stroke is required. It's true that coconut oil—and palm oil—are saturated. However, not all saturated oils are processed by your body in the same way (see box below). Coconut contains a couple types of fats that are very protective against viruses, bacteria, and other pathogens. In fact, these same fats are an important component of the breast milk of nursing mothers that gives infants immunity against illness.

ALL FATS ARE NOT CREATED EQUAL

Fats come in different length chains, similar to a beaded necklace. There are long-chain, medium-chain, and short-chain fatty acids. Short- and medium-chain fatty acids are digested relatively easily and can then be used by the body for energy. But remember that your body can only use a certain amount of energy and then excess calories will be turned into fat. So if your body doesn't need the energy from fat, it will be stored as fat rather than burned. If your body has been flooded with too many calories of carbohydrate energy (glucose), it will also not be able to utilize this fat.

Coconut oil and the fat in coconut meat are short- and medium-chain fatty acids your body can burn; the fact that they are saturated fats does not make them more likely to be stored in your arteries.

OUT WITH THE BAD FATS

Go through your cabinets, refrigerator, and freezer and read package labels, looking for food that has hydrogenated or partially hydrogenated vegetable oils. Decide if you want to throw them out; or, if that feels too wasteful to you, phase them out of your diet as you use them up. (Please do consider the cost to your health as well as your food budget.) Begin looking carefully at package labels as you shop. *Anything* that is not a fresh, whole food in a raw state is a possible candidate for harboring these health-damaging, manufactured fats.

IN WITH THE GOOD

Shop for a variety of healthy fat sources to begin including in your diet. Remember that healthy fat can be added with foods as well as oils. Coconut, nuts, peanut or almond butter, sesame tahini, olives, and avocados can all be included in small amounts as part of your meals and snacks. Olive oil, sesame oil, and coconut oil can be used for stir-fry cooking. Olive oil and flaxseed oil together make great salad dressings. Use the "Fish Sources of Omega 3 Fatty Acids" list on page 42 to select fish for at least two meals a week. Look through the recipes at the back to see how healthy fats can be incorporated into your meals

PRACTICAL TIPS FOR INCLUDING HEALTHY FAT

In general, heating decreases the amount and digestibility of nutrients in fat. This means most of your added fat intake should be in the cold, raw form. Think about getting most of your fat from those naturally occurring in whole foods, such as nuts, seeds, nut butters, sesame tahini, olives, avocados, and foods made from these items. The majority of the oil you use should be in raw form as well as sauces, marinades, or salad dressings. The Cookbook section contains many such recipes. The natural fats in meat, fish, dairy products, vegetables, and grains will meet the remainder of your fat needs. The more fat you take in from meat, fish, and dairy, the less added fat you need, and vice versa.

Selection and Storage

Look for extra virgin olive oil. For other vegetable and seed oils, look for the words "cold pressed" or "expellar pressed" on the label. Oils should be in a dark-colored or lightproof container. Because it contains natural antioxidants, olive oil can keep well at room temperature, but should be kept away from light, and, in hot weather, kept in a cool place. Other vegetable or seed oils should be refrigerated. Olive, sesame, walnut, coconut, and flaxseed oils will meet most needs.

Cooking

The best oils for sautéing are olive oil, sesame oil, or coconut oil. A blend of equal parts of all three can be used as well. Coconut and sesame oils are more stable than other oils when heated.

Baking

Remember, in healing nutrition you want to minimize your use of refined flours and sweeteners. This means, in large part, redefining "treats" and creating desserts that don't rely on typical baking ingredients, i.e., flour, sugar, etc. (Chapter Ten will help you do this.) Having said that, though, if you were going to bake something, the best fats to use would be solid ones, such as butter or coconut oil, which are solid at room temperature. Solid fats perform better in baking and both of these fats have the benefit of providing several antimicrobial fatty acids that protect and promote health.

Mayonnaise

The ideal mayonnaise to use would be made from olive oil. Since this is almost impossible to find ready-made in the store, the next best thing would be to find a safflower or canola oil mayonnaise made from cold pressed or expeller pressed oil, available in a health food store. This processing is far less damaging than most commercial versions of the same oils. One such brand is Spectrum Natural®, which comes in both a regular and light version.

Sauces, Dressings

Olive oil, flaxseed oil, sesame tahini, sesame oil, and the nut butters can be used to make interesting and delicious sauces, vegetable toppings, marinades, and salad dressings. Even though these are healthy fat sources, don't forget that you still need to monitor the amount of fat you take in!

FATS THAT PROMOTE HEALTH

1) **Naturally occurring saturated fats** found in grass-fed meat, hormone-free dairy products, and coconut oil

2) **Omega 9 monounsaturated fats,** such as those found in olive oil, avocado, nuts, and seeds

3) **Omega 3** found in fish, flaxseed, and flaxseed oil

4) **Omega 6 polyunsaturated fats** naturally occurring in vegetables and grains.

(Most of these foods contain more than one of the Omega fats; they are listed by the fat that is most predominant.)

HOW MUCH IS ENOUGH?

Fat intake varies widely in different parts of the world. The general range is anywhere from 10 percent to more than 50 percent of calories from fat. Needs vary depending on energy requirements, climate, and health. In the United States and Canada, government food guidelines and health association guidelines for fat intake are similar—roughly 30 percent of calories from fat. In following these guidelines, the most important factor is the kind and quality of fat you are consuming. If you are eating 30 percent of your calories from fat, approximately 25 percent of your daily calories should come from the Omega 3 and 9 fats (saturated and monosaturated) combined, and 5 percent from Omega 6 (polyunsaturated) sources. Since the Omega 6 fats are present in so many food sources and in most Omega 3 and 9 fats, you don't need to add Omega 6 fats to your diet.

In my practice, I have found the 30 percent number is somewhat arbitrary. What seems to be more significant is:

1) the source of the fat
2) that the overall caloric need is not exceeded

I recommend that clients keep their saturated fat level to 10 to12 percent of overall calories and make all additional fat come from the Omega 3 and 9 categories, meaning fish, nuts, nut butters, olive oil, olives, avocado, flaxseed meal, and flaxseed oil. Many of my clients exceed the 30 percent number but do observe the two guidelines above. Because fat is more satisfying, it helps you eat less. Combined with controlling carbohydrates, a moderate rather than a low-fat diet helps improve overall physical and emotional health.

In Chapter Three you will learn more about how to translate fat percentages into more practical measures of food.

CHILDREN AND FAT

Even before birth, a growing fetus needs a good supply of healthy fat. German research shows that trans-fatty acids consumed by the mother are a factor in low birth weight and also interfere with DHA formation in the brain. Trans-fatty acids consumed by a lactating mother go directly into her breast milk. Canadian research shows that these fats are correlated with a decreased visual acuity in infants.

Breast milk contains over 50 percent fat, over 25 percent of which is saturated. The infant brain needs this fat for proper development. Cholesterol is very important in the visual development of children. A very young child (birth to two years) needs 50 percent of calories from *healthy fats.* If you feel a need to decrease the fat content of your child's diet to conform to the 30 percent guideline, do it gradually, reaching 30 percent at the age of eighteen, when primary growth and development ends. Greasy fast food, hydrogenated fats in prepackaged snack food, and baked goods interfere with the physical, emotional, and mental balance in kids.

Remember This...

Saturated animal fat in meat, eggs, dairy food, and butter in moderate quantities is not inherently bad for you. Highly refined vegetable oils, the kind most often used in commercially packaged and restaurant-prepared food, are the most harmful to health because they are:

1) oxidized, promoting free-radical activity and damage in your body
2) chemically altered to form trans-fatty acids, which interfere with your body's use of health-promoting, essential fatty acids

USING FLAXSEED OIL

In general I recommend a baseline for flaxseed oil of one to two tablespoons/ day for restoring and building health. Some people find this easiest to accomplish by taking eight 1,000mg capsules (equivalent to one tablespoon), and then whatever extra that comes from food is a bonus. Two tablespoons of ground flax meal is equivalent to ½ teaspoon of the oil.

Some health benefits of using flaxseed oil regularly are:

- Softer, more supple skin, relief of skin conditions such as eczema, psoriasis
- Reduced pain and inflammation from conditions such as arthritis, lupus, and fibromyalgia
- Reduced risk of stroke, heart disease, and cancer
- Better ability to metabolize fat
- Better thyroid regulation
- Lower LDL ("bad") cholesterol
- Higher HDL ("good") cholesterol

Ways to incorporate flaxseed oil and meal into your diet:

- Add 1 tablespoon flax meal or 1 teaspoon to 1 tablespoon flaxseed oil to smoothies
- Drizzle a teaspoon of oil over steamed vegetables
- Use flaxseed oil in oatmeal instead of butter or top with flax meal
- Substitute for half or all of the olive oil in salad dressings (uncooked only)
- Use ground flaxseed on top of oatmeal or as a topping on yogurt with fruit or fruit cobblers

Selecting and storing flaxseed oil, flax seeds, or flax meal:

- Should be stored in refrigerator (in the health store as well)
- Buy only in opaque (lightproof) containers to protect from light
- Purchase what you will use in about three months' time
- Extra may be stored in freezer for six months
- Make sure oil is unrefined, unprocessed, and organic if possible
- Heating will destroy oil; use raw (flax meal can tolerate some heat)
- If using flaxseeds, store in freezer and grind enough for several days only
- Buying ground flax meal is convenient, but it loses potency more quickly

EVALUATING YOUR DIETARY FAT

Go over your food journals for a week and see if you can determine the sources of your dietary fat.

Healthy:
- Meat, Poultry, Dairy, Eggs, Butter, Coconut Oil
- Nuts, Seeds, Nut Butters, Olives, Olive Oil, Avocado, Nut and Seed Oils (walnut, sesame, etc.)
- Fish, Flaxseed, Flaxseed Oil

Unhealthy:
- Margarine
- Commercial (not cold-pressed nor organic) vegetable oils
- Hydrogenated or partially hydrogenated fats in prepackaged foods

You can be sure that, unless stated otherwise, most restaurants will use commercial vegetable oils and foods that contain hydrogenated fat, such as prepared dressings or commercially baked breads, rolls, and crackers. Restaurants that prepare their own dressings should have at least one olive oil-based dressing that contains only healthy fat.

MOVING FORWARD

Whether you succeed or fail at any venture depends in large part on whether you believe you can succeed and are deserving of success. This is true in every area of your life. In the previous chapter you were asked to write down your goals and also to make a list of negative thoughts and any beliefs or attitudes you feel might get in the way of meeting your health goals. If you have not done that, you need to complete those tasks to work with the exercises in this chapter that focus on getting your subconscious mind to cooperate in meeting your health goals.

HOW THE SUBCONSCIOUS WORKS

Your subconscious doesn't much care whether it plays a chorus for you of self-defeating or of positive messages. It will do whatever it has been "programmed" to do. So if you have found in the past that you have not been successful with your efforts to change how you eat or to incorporate exercise routines into your life or to achieve any other goal, the reason may be that you don't really believe you can do it. Having a subconscious that echoes positive messages is like having a good friend by your side who always says, "I know you can do this," "Way to go," "You are going to reach your goals." Couldn't we all use that kind of encouragement and motivation?

Two things impress the subconscious:
1) repetition
2) emotion

The idea that we won't succeed at changing usually is linked to having heard repeated suggestions earlier in life, that we aren't up to snuff in one way or another. Frequently those kinds of messages were made at moments that were highly emotionally charged. This combination leaves one with self-limiting images and beliefs about the self. Are you aware of where your critical messages and limiting beliefs and attitudes originated? Whether you are or not, you still can change them. Using the same characteristics of repetition and emotion, you can get your subconscious to give you positive instead of self-sabotaging thoughts and images.

A positive statement made to you with energy and enthusiasm, over and over again, can cause your perceptions of and beliefs about yourself to change. And that, in turn, prompts you to take different actions, which help you move closer to your goals. But it would be simplistic to think if you just start saying "I will be healthy" enthusiastically, over and over again, your life is going to change. Let's talk a little more about how to effectively get your subconscious working for you.

POSITIVE AFFIRMATIONS AND VISUALIZATIONS

There are five characteristics of positive affirmations and visualizations that make them effective. They must be:

1) **personal**   4) **positive**
2) **precise**   5) **persistent**
3) **present**

Personal: This one I think is reasonably obvious; *you* need to be the object of the affirmation. If your goal is to make healthy food choices when you eat at restaurants, for example, you wouldn't want an affirmation stating "My coworkers won't pressure me into eating desserts." An affirmation needs to have "I" at the center of it. "I am making *great* choices for myself every time I go out to eat" would be an example of making the affirmation personal.

Precise: Precision is very important. To be successful, we have to develop and hold a clear and precise vision of how it is we want to be. People who are successful have a capacity to see themselves as they want to be, and it's that vision that leads them to their goals. How easily are you able to create pictures, think of concepts, hear sounds, and feel sensations that go along with your goals? Filling in as much sensory detail about how you want to be is important. Maybe you've been there before and can supply the detail from memory. If not, it comes from imagination or seeing someone else who "has what you want."

If you're not someone who easily creates mental pictures, don't let that stop you. Not everyone uses the sensory channel of sight as a primary sensory mode. If your sense of hearing or sensation is stronger, create your successful story in that sense. Do try however, to make your "picture" as multisensorial as you possibly can.

Let's look at some examples. If your goal is to lose weight, a more precise goal would be to pick an item of clothing or an outfit that you want to be able to wear. Then you can create a detailed sensory experience of what you look and feel like in that clothing. Or your goal might be to initiate and maintain a power-walking program. See yourself doing that activity; hear the sounds that go along with it, feel your body going through the motions.

Filling in the sensory details of living as though you had already attained your goals may not come naturally to you. It may feel foreign or even scary to do that. It's a learned skill that takes practice. When I first conceived of writing this book, I knew I had the knowledge, desire, and skill to write it, but, frankly, as much as I talked about doing it, I never quite had the conviction that I would actually accomplish it. It was only when I began to see myself writing it that I created the space in my life to do it. How many goals do you have that you truly want but can't really imagine yourself reaching?

Imagining yourself being successful in full, living color doesn't mean pretending the reality of your present circumstances do not exist. It just means that you are willing to see other possibilities. And if you can see them, you can realize them. If you can't, you won't.

Present: The subconscious doesn't differentiate past, present, and future. Everything is now. So get rid of ambiguous references, such as "I will be able to walk five miles next June" and give your mind the message "I am walking five miles." Your subconscious will accept any idea as true as long as it is impressed with the feeling of reality. You can accomplish this best by staying in the present tense with your words and your visualizations.

Positive: The subconscious does not process negative words like "not," "can't," or "won't." It just filters them out. It's difficult to visualize *not* doing "x" or "y." When you give yourself a message of "I won't eat chocolate when I feel stressed," the image you are left with is one of eating chocolate. If there's some behavior you'd like to stop doing, figure out what is the positive behavior you want to do in its place and create your affirmation based on doing the positive behavior, such as "When I'm under stress I take ten deep breaths." Then your brain can hold an image of you engaging in the desired behavior.

I had a very clear demonstration of that principle in my life. I am a defensive player on a women's ice hockey team. One of my jobs is to keep the puck away from the goal, and when it comes in front of my team's goal, I am supposed to hit it toward the sideboards of the rink. During one game, the puck came to me and I hit it up the middle of the ice, allowing the other team's player to get a clear shot on goal. When I got off the ice, my coach said to me, "Don't hit it up the middle." I repeated to myself, "Not up the middle, not up the middle." My next shift on the ice, I did the exact same thing with the puck. My coach just shook his head. My third shift out, I told myself even more firmly, "Okay, you're not going to hit it up the middle." Well you can guess what happened that time, can't you? It wasn't until I changed what I was telling myself, and what I visualized, that my reaction on the ice changed. I switched to "I am hitting the puck to the sideboards" and I saw myself doing it, felt myself doing it. I immediately stopped making the mistake of passing the puck up the middle.

Persistent: This refers to the aspect of repetition we discussed earlier. Once you have your goal written as an "I" statement, in the present tense, with full sensory detail, using only positive language, repeat it over and over to yourself. Say it out loud, no matter how silly you feel. Say it silently to yourself. Write it on a piece of paper and place the paper somewhere private if you wish, but somewhere you'll see it often. Repeat, repeat, repeat. When you wake up, when you're in the shower or in the car, while you're walking, just before you fall asleep, take a few minutes and repeat your affirmations either out loud or to yourself. Allow yourself to imagine your goal as if it were happening *in that moment*. Doing this on a regular basis will increase your success.

 RELAXATION

There is one other factor that helps to turn your affirmations and visualizations into action and reality: relaxation. There is a simple reason for this. Your subconscious is more receptive when you are relaxed.

You can increase your success by getting yourself into a relaxed state before you work with your affirmations and visualizations. A wide selection of tapes are available designed to help you relax. Here are some guidelines to help you, with or without music.

1. Find a time when you have fifteen to twenty minutes during which you won't be interrupted.

2. Get comfortable; sit or lie down and loosen any restrictive clothing.

3. Take several deep breaths in through the nose, hold a few seconds, and exhale slowly through your mouth. Focus on feeling your breath fill your entire body, then empty from it.

4. Tell yourself, "I am relaxing," "My body is sinking into the couch (chair)," "My pulse is slowing down," "I am letting go of all tension," etc.

5. After about five minutes of getting into a relaxed state, begin repeating your affirmations with as much feeling and authenticity as you can. Also, give yourself time to see, hear, and feel yourself doing whatever your goal is. Continue this process for about ten minutes. You may feel silly at first, but just have fun with it!

6. When you are ready to end, slowly count backward from five to one. With each number, feel yourself becoming more conscious of your physical surroundings, your body, and the present moment.

If you can impress upon your subconscious mind the feeling of reality about your goals, it will work on validating your affirmations and visualizations.

INTERRUPTING NEGATIVE THOUGHTS

Maybe right now you're thinking to yourself, "Yeah, this sounds good on paper, but I just can't believe something that is so far from reality." Maybe you've tried to use positive affirmations before and negative thoughts and self-doubts hounded you. This is very common. And, there is a process for stamping out these intrusive naysayers. It's a very simple process. Whenever a negative thought about reaching your goal comes out of your mouth or enters your mind, simply say in a very strong voice, preferably out loud, "CANCEL!" What you are trying to do is make a distinct impression on your subconscious by using strong emotion in conjunction with the statement "Cancel." Thinking that you won't succeed at something you would like to accomplish is a habit. And, like any other habit, it can be changed with focused effort.

STAMPING OUT NEGATIVE MESSAGES

Use the list of negative thoughts, beliefs, and attitudes you wrote for Moving Forward in Chapter One. Bring yourself into a relaxed state using the procedure above. Before you begin doing any positive affirmations or visualizations, imagine that all your negative messages are written on a big screen in front of you. Then, as you're seeing them, loudly say, "CANCEL," "CANCEL," "CANCEL" three times. At the same time, see all the writing disappear, going up into a cloud of smoke. Then proceed with your affirmations and visualizations.

CONSCIOUSLY CHOOSING TO SUCCEED

This week take the goals that you wrote for yourself and rewrite them as positive affirmations, making sure they are personal, precise, present, and positive. Spend time imagining yourself successfully achieving your goals in as much sensory detail as you can. Then, use the affirmations and visualizations persistently! See the sample affirmations below.

- Try doing the relaxation exercise with your affirmations and visualizations. The more frequently you can make time for this, the more likely and the quicker your success will be.

- Practice interrupting negative thinking. Use your list of negative thoughts, beliefs, and attitudes to do the visualization exercise of canceling negative thoughts.

Here are some samples of positive affirmations regarding healthy eating and a healthy body:

I have a healthy body and I enjoy walking every day.
I love feeding my body healthy food!
I look fabulous in my _____(article of clothing)!
I enjoy feeling lighter and moving with ease.

I am controlling my blood sugar with great food choices.

I am packing myself healthy meals and snacks to take to work.

In May, I am walking a 5K race. (Note that even though a future date is named, the affirmation is in the present.)

Healthy food tastes delicious to me; I prefer it to junk food.

I eat when my body tells me I am hungry.

I love and appreciate my healthy body.

I walk three flights of stairs with plenty of energy and ease.

NOW, WHAT
ARE **YOUR** GOALS AND
AFFIRMATIONS?

CHAPTER THREE

GOOD MEALS, GOOD MOOD

Today, more than ever, people are suffering from a range of difficulties relating to both mood and mental functioning. Mood and mind-altering medications are prescribed with alarming frequency, and children are increasingly among those being treated with potent and frequently highly addictive psychiatric drugs.

Depression, anxiety, attention deficit disorder, mental fatigue, inability to concentrate, difficulty with problem solving and decisionmaking, poor memory, frequent irritability, and Jeckyll and Hyde mood swings are common complaints today. Not all of these symptoms lead people to seek medication but for many they interfere with school, work, relationships, and family life.

What many of these symptoms have in common is that they frequently originate in a biochemical imbalance in the brain. In some individuals, a genetic or organic predisposition to the imbalance may exist; in others, not. However, in both groups of people, nutrition is a highly effective means of restoring the proper balance in brain chemistry. Food you eat is a significant factor in how the brain functions. So important is diet, that many people find maintaining a well-planned diet can take the place of mood-altering medication. While not everybody is able to regulate brain-chemical imbalances through diet alone, even those who still require pharmaceutical support will be helped by developing good eating habits, as good nutrition can stabilize brain chemistry.

"Good Meals, Good Moods" will explore some of the food choices you can make to optimize your mental functioning and improve your emotional well-being.

UNDERSTANDING YOUR BODY

MOOD, MENTAL PROCESSES, & YOUR BRAIN'S CHEMICAL SOUP

Today, we have a more sophisticated understanding of brain chemicals and mood than ever before. Although life situations play a big part in mood, mood changes, and mental processes, *neurotransmitters* are the physical agents of mental and emotional changes. Like little emails travelling through the Internet, five basic neurotransmitters carry information to "mailboxes," called "receptor sites," throughout your brain and body.

1. **Serotonin**—This natural chemical stabilizes mood, increases your ability to focus and thoughtfully solve problems, controls impulsiveness, and creates a general sense of optimism and well-being. Serotonin also helps promote sleep.

2. **Beta-Endorphin**—These are the body's natural painkillers on both the emotional and physical levels. They raise our threshold for physical discomfort and pain. The more beta-endorphin you have, the less likely you are to overreact to criticism or to someone else's sad story. Empathy is one thing; not being able to emotionally separate from someone else's troubles is often due to a beta-endorphin shortage. Beta-endorphin is also largely responsible for feelings of self-esteem; the more beta-endorphin the brain makes, the higher one's feelings of self-esteem, and vice versa.

3. & 4. Dopamine and Norepinephrine—These two brain chemicals provide energy, alertness, drive, and mental focus.

5.   **GABA** (gamma amino butyric acid)—GABA is a natural sedative, providing a sense of calm, relaxation, and relief from anxiety. It also provides relaxation in your gut, helping to prevent ulcers and irritable bowel-type symptoms.

Many people do not have enough of one or more of these brain chemicals. Depending on the type of imbalance a person has, their difficulties with mood and mental functioning will vary. Sometimes a person is genetically predisposed to a neurochemical imbalance. That doesn't mean he or she absolutely will have one; but if a person is predisposed, poor nutrition and high levels of stress are more likely to result in an imbalance. Many times, stress and a nutrition imbalance alone will result in a person having too little of one or more neurotransmitters. Sometimes a diet lacks the food necessary to create the neurotransmitters, or to build and maintain the "information superhighway" they travel along. Sometimes it's a substance such as caffeine that can destroy a particular neurotransmitter (such as GABA), leaving the brain and body at a deficit.

In my twenty years of practicing as a psychotherapist, I found that many emotions and behaviors typically considered "grist for the therapy mill" in fact were often more connected to a client's biochemistry and largely affected by diet. Sometimes, three weeks of dietary change could produce more change than three years of psychotherapy! Though not everybody experiences such dramatic changes, changing one's diet certainly will contribute to an improved ability to think clearly, stay alert and focused, handle stress, and feel a general sense of optimism. And, mood-supporting nutrition can greatly enhance personal-growth work.

Each of the neurotransmitters is manufactured in the brain from amino acids. There is only one dietary source for amino acids, and that is protein. Each neurotransmitter has a different amino acid precursor, meaning an amino acid that is converted into the specific brain chemical. In addition, endorphin release is stimulated through exercise and other activities that involve energy movement in the body. Yoga, singing, laughter, meditation, prayer, and sex are all examples of activities that stimulate endorphin production and release.

Although there are a number of reasons a person might not have enough of one or more neurotransmitters, a common one, and the one we all have the most control over, is lack of a sufficient amount of protein. Eating more protein will provide more amino acids precursors to be converted.

Figuring out which protein source will provide the necessary kind of amino acids is not complicated. All protein from animal sources is what we call "complete," meaning it contains all twenty-two amino acids the body requires. Nine of these amino acids are considered essential, because the body cannot manufacture them on its own. Vegetarian protein sources, with the exception of soy, are called "incomplete," because they are missing one or more of the essential amino acids. But soy protein, while also complete, contains a substance that interferes with protein metabolism, called trypsin inhibitor. If you are vegetarian, your diet needs to include a variety of plant sources to combine and provide all the required amino acids. You don't have to combine them all in the same meal, but over the course of a day.

Eating protein throughout the day, at meals and for snacks, will provide your body with the ingredients it needs to keep your transmitters in good supply. I have never had a client who didn't respond to eating more protein by having more energy, a better mental focus, and an improved mood.

People who are short on the basic neurotransmitters tend to crave sugary and quickly dissolving (refined) carbohydrate foods. These foods temporarily relieve some of the discomfort of having too few of the basic neurotransmitters. Refined carbohydrates cause a temporary increase in serotonin, endorphin-like effect, and energy. For a short period of time, one might feel happier, more alert, and energetic, but the effect is short-lived. Ultimately, eating this way will result in more depletion, more depression, lethargy, and decreased mental acuity. And it's easy to get caught in an endless cycle of craving refined foods, feeling better then worse, craving more of the wrong foods, etc.

Below, we will consider some of the other imbalances that play a role in problems with mood and mental functioning.

DEPRESSION, HYPOGLYCEMIA, AND SUGAR SENSITIVITY

In Chapter One, we discussed some of the symptoms of hypoglycemia, many of which have to do with mood and mental functioning. Mood swings, irritability, memory loss, confused thinking, and an inability to focus can all result when blood-sugar levels drop. The person then gets caught in the vicious craving cycle described above. A diet high in refined carbohydrates and sugar is frequently behind chronic depression and decreased mental functioning; eating a lot of these foods usually makes one feel lethargic and without much energy or motivation for moving and exercising. Naturally, in addition to depression, this lifestyle leads to weight gain as well, usually compounding the depression. Eliminating these foods from the diet will produce surprising and desirable changes in mood and outlook as well as physical health. Parents who institute these changes in the diets of their children frequently find they have a more cooperative child with an agreeable disposition. One mother told me about a dramatic change that happened after making these changes in her family's diet. Her son began doing his homework after school with no prodding from her! Previously each day had been marked by arguments and struggles that dragged on from afternoon into evening as she tried to get her son to do his studying.

Some people who struggle with depression are more sensitive to ups and downs in blood sugar. Their bodies have higher highs and lower lows in response to refined carbohydrates. These folks have the misfortune of a chemistry that is predisposed both to a shortage of neurotransmitters *and* hypoglycemia. This double imbalance, which is quite common, exerts a stronger pull on the person to eat refined carbohydrates. These cravings are not the result of a weak will, but of a misguided, unconscious effort to feel better.

Here are some of the characteristics that often signal this increased sensitivity to refined carbohydrates:

- Strong cravings for sweets, starchy carbohydrates, or both
- Parents who had this kind of diet or craving
- Personal or family history of excessive alcohol or substance use
- An inability to lose excess weight
- Chronic or frequent bouts of depression
- Sneaking food or being secretive or private about eating
- Family history of depression

How many of these characteristics describe you?

If you suffer from depression, I strongly encourage you to look at your diet, particularly if you find several of the above characteristics apply to you. Oftentimes, a person will begin taking a prescription antidepressant without changing his or her diet. I find that the antidepressant is less effective if the person is still eating a lot of refined carbohydrates. Although the drug may seem to help, the ups and downs in blood sugar still have a negative effect on mood. I have also worked with many people who changed their diets and eliminated their depression without the use of prescription medication.

TINA was a forty-four-year-old woman who came to see me because she wanted to stop eating sugar and believed that would help with her irritable bowel and diverticulitis. As we talked she let me know that she struggled with depression, was frequently anxious, and had a family history of depression. Her anxiety took the form of her being extremely self-conscious when she was with other people, always monitoring what she was saying and doing and watching for other's reactions. She also tended to get stuck in her thinking, turning the same problem over and over again in her mind. She liked exercise and participated in dance classes but wanted to increase her activity level. She also told me that she didn't know much about cooking and that planning meals was difficult for her.

Her diet consisted primarily of fast food, candy, cookies, frozen waffles, and popcorn, punctuated by a serving of meat about once a day and a vegetable a few times a week. We worked together for six months, helping her add protein, vegetables, and healthy fat and to eliminate most sugar and refined carbohydrates. I was able to help her with menu planning, shopping, and developing some cooking and kitchen organizational skills. She also learned how to satisfy her sweet tooth in healthy ways.

Tina's story is one of the most dramatic instances I've seen of dietary changes producing physical and emotional changes, partly because she was so motivated and committed to making those changes. Tina did not want to use mood-altering medication to break out of the family pattern of depression and anxiety. She also wanted to handle her irritable bowel problems naturally and address the underlying problem, not just medicate the symptoms.

Over the course of the six months, I watched as Tina's depression lifted, her anxiety disappeared in all but the most stressful situations, and she became more outgoing and comfortable socially. All of her irritable bowel symptoms disappeared and her blood pressure, which had been elevated, dropped to normal. Most of these changes happened within the first two months and the benefits simply solidified or increased as time went on. By the end of the six months, she was adept at planning and cooking food to carry her through her busy weeks, with a minimal amount of time spent in the kitchen. Most important, she was no longer depressed, was infrequently troubled by anxiety, and had the energy and ease to add new interests and friends to her life.

REFINED CARBOHYDRATES AND ALCOHOLISM

Because of the predisposition to a neurochemical imbalance, some people are drawn to alcohol or substance abuse for much the same reasons people are drawn to sugar and refined foods. Alcohol and drugs provide the same temporary relief from the discomfort of the biochemical imbalances. When I worked as a therapist in an inpatient substance abuse program, sugar-laden desserts and starchy carbohydrate food was the standard fare of the hospital's dietary service, and the clients loved it. Of course they did! It provided some of the relief they were no longer getting from drugs or alcohol. Unfortunately, such a diet keeps the cravings for drugs and alcohol alive and makes the recovering alcoholic or drug user very vulnerable to a relapse. In a few forward-thinking programs around the country, nutrition is being used as part of the rehabilitation process. The long-term success rate in those programs that restrict sugar and refined carbohydrates is around 80 percent, compared to 20 or 25 percent in standard treatment programs.

If you have either a family or a personal history that includes overuse of alcohol or drugs, past or present, following the dietary guidelines in this program will greatly improve your chances for long-term sobriety.

BALANCING MOODS WITH MEALS

By now, it should be clear that refined carbohydrates serve neither your brain nor your body, and that eating them only creates cravings for more of them. Natural, unprocessed, fiber-rich carbohydrates from the vegetable, fruit, grain, and legume families are the carbohydrate choices that will provide adequate fuel for your muscles and brain. Combine these with regular, sufficient amounts of protein and your brain will have the ingredients it needs to manufacture the neurotransmitters responsible for keeping you optimistic, calm, alert, motivated, able to concentrate, and thinking clearly.

In Chapter Two, you learned how important sufficient quantities of healthy fats are in the formation of your brain and nervous system. If the brain and nervous system are structurally compromised, they are unable to make optimal use of the neurotransmitters, even if the brain is producing them in sufficient quantities.

Nerve endings require the essential fatty acids from the natural polyunsaturated fats, particularly the essential fat known as *Decosahexanoic Acid or DHA*. Eighty percent of the material in nerve endings should be DHA, a fat occurring naturally only in fish. Whenever there is insufficient DHA, other fats fill the void. Often the fats that fill in are the unhealthy, manufactured fats that are so prevalent in our diets today. These fats negatively affect how efficiently the nerve cells transmit the information provided by the neurotransmitters by slowing down the firing process.

Your body is able to make DHA from other natural polyunsaturates, the Omega 3 fatty acids such as flaxseed, or evening primrose oil, but this conversion is not very efficient. It is estimated that we can convert only about 10 percent of these plant-based Omega 3 fatty acids to DHA. Several things can interfere with this conversion, including hydrogenated or trans-fats in the diet. Polyunsaturated vegetable oils like cottonseed, corn, soy, safflower, canola, and sunflower that are high in Omega 6 fatty acids can also interfere with this conversion. These fats and oils compete with or depress the enzymes necessary to make the conversion to DHA. Also, people with certain metabolic diseases like diabetes may have problems making the conversion to DHA. For all these reasons it is best to make sure you have enough DHA by including it in your diet through either fish or fish oil supplements.

The National Institutes of Health are now conducting many studies into the effectiveness of Omega 3 fatty acids in the treatment of bipolar disorder, kidney disease, cancer (specifically its relationship to weight loss), and cardiovascular disease. A preliminary study conducted by Harvard University researchers demonstrated that fish oil has significant mood-stabilizing effects for those suffering from bipolar disorder.[1]

So you can see how inadequate healthy fat or too much unhealthy fat in the diet ultimately plays a very big role in mental and emotional health.

Does this all seem complicated? It doesn't have to be. Even if you don't follow the chemistry and physiology, it all boils down to this:

- Adequate protein
- High-quality carbohydrates
- Adequate healthy fats
- Avoiding processed carbohydrates and sugary foods
- Avoiding manufactured fats

By now, you hopefully have developed or are working on the habit of eating protein throughout the day. If you need to, go back to the Nutrition Magic sections of Chapters One and Two and review healthy protein choices and healthy fat choices. In this Nutrition Magic section you will learn more about combining protein, fat, and carbohydrate for optimal health. You will

[1] Stoll et al, *Archives of General Psychiatry*, December 1999, 56:407-412

also be able to determine an overall dietary approach to fit your health needs. And if you are nervous that reducing or eliminating sugar means never having a sweet treat again, fear not! In Chapter Ten you'll learn about alternative sweeteners that won't throw off your brain and body chemistry. Then be sure to peruse the Sweet Treat recipe section at the back of the book.

Exercise is one of the most effective ways of improving both mood and physical health. In this chapter's Moving Forward section, we'll look at how and why exercise can help you feel better.

NUTRITION MAGIC

Every bite you take is a choice you make about how well you care for yourself.

CREATING A PERSONAL DIETARY ROADMAP

Like you perhaps, I have read and tried just about every diet plan for weight loss or health. Most work initially because the dieter suddenly becomes more conscious of what he or she is eating. Sometimes diets work because they break the body of a routine, and just doing something different seems to shake things up a bit. But most plans either focus exclusively on restricting calories or are extreme diets that are unlikely to be sustained for any extended period of time. Most assume that everyone has the same health and nutrition needs. *Take Two Apples and Call Me in the Morning* is not a "one plan fits all" approach to nutrition and health. But you have to be willing to give up the idea that there is a single diet out there that offers you a magic bullet—there isn't. Are you prepared to do that?

Finding the nutritional style that works for you involves your participation. Most of us are used to the model of a "diet." A diet is someone else's idea of a specific regimen to be followed to produce a desired result—often, but not exclusively, weight reduction. In this program, you are learning about what your body and brain need to function optimally. You are learning how different foods can either enhance or detract from health. And, you are learning to pay attention to how *you* respond to eating different foods.

What you will find here is a summary of the guiding principles that we've developed so far for you to use in planning your meals and snacks. Following that summary are three plans, each with a sample menu. One of these plans is likely to fit your present needs. Each menu is slightly different in meal composition as far as the quantities of protein, carbohydrate, and fat, and each has some notes about who might benefit from such a menu and why. I've also given examples of typical client notes from my clinical practice. You will see actual client food logs from their first visit, followed by the initial steps I recommended based on 1) the client's health needs, and 2) their established eating patterns. These demonstrate more realistically the *process* of changing your diet.

> Changing how you eat doesn't happen because someone gives you a piece of paper with the "right" foods written on it. It happens because each day you think, plan, make choices, and take one more step in the direction of better health. Some days you step backwards. Investing in your health is like investing in the stock market; it's best if you recognize that you're in it for the long haul.

You will have the most success if you create a plan, then faithfully carry it out for a few months, all the while observing and logging how you feel, and noting any changes in energy, mood, weight, blood chemistry, etc. Be aware that if you've been eating a lot of carbohydrates, it generally takes a few months for your body's metabolism to shift so it can consistently burn fat more efficiently. On the other hand, I have many diabetic clients who report blood-sugar normalization within three days to two weeks. Energy levels and mood changes can occur in an equally short amount of time. If you don't notice changes that quickly, be patient. Often healing is happening at a deeper level in your body and the changes may not be readily apparent. Sometimes you may feel temporarily worse as your body and mind "withdraw" from sugar or refined carbohydrates. Everyone will be different in how long it takes him or her to get new habits into place. It's important to give yourself a fair trial, and to be honest with yourself about how consistently you are practicing your new habits.

Your nutritional needs change as your health changes, as you increase your activity level, as you age, and as the seasons change. Although this program outlines some basic principles of nutrition and wellness, once again I want to remind you that this program is not a diet. *Take Two Apples* is a tool kit, and I invite you to become more skilled as you practice using its tools. You are the best health care provider you have!

OLD VERSUS NEW WAYS OF THINKING

First let's review some of the new ways of thinking you have learned about in Chapters One and Two.

OLD THINKING	NEW THINKING
• The old way concerns restricting how much you eat.	• The new way focuses on the food quality and eating regularly. While calories do matter, restricted-calorie diets accommodate a sluggish metabolism instead of helping it burn calories and fat more efficiently, which is our focus. You begin eliminating foods that slow down metabolism and increase foods that speed it up.
• The old way is "anything goes as long as it's low-fat."	• The new way looks at food's impact on blood sugar and insulin regulation. We control blood sugar by eliminating or strictly limiting use of white flour-based products, limiting use of refined-grain products in general (e.g., wheat flour, cereals, cornmeal), and eliminating or strictly limiting use of sugar and other concentrated sweeteners. *Natural* sweeteners are preferable to low-fat.

OLD THINKING	NEW THINKING
• The old way of thinking is that carbohydrates are "good" because they provide energy, nutrients, and are low in fat.	• The new way evaluates carbohydrates individually for their healthfulness. The more processed they are, the higher their impact on blood sugar and insulin, and the more likely they are to stimulate fat storage, overeating, fatigue, mood changes, and elevated cholesterol. We choose carbohydrates that are high in fiber, are minimally altered from their natural state, and provide energy without creating highs and lows in blood sugar.
• The old way is that saturated fat and cholesterol are bad, no-cholesterol vegetable oils and margarine are good.	• The new way recognizes some saturated fat and cholesterol is vital for good health, and in moderate amounts these are far less harmful to health than manufactured fats and oils. The natural mono- and polyunsaturated fats found in fish, nuts, seeds, olives, avocados, flax, and vegetables are extremely beneficial to health.
• The old way is that there is one correct way of eating (even though nobody seems to agree on what that is).	• The new way acknowledges that each person needs to adjust diet to fit his or her current circumstances.

Next, let's apply some overall guiding principles:

1. Eat regularly throughout the day, tapering off after sunset (unless you work or are physically active at night). Your metabolism slows down naturally with nightfall as your body prepares for restorative and repair work.

2. Avoid white flour, white sugar, and products made from them. Limit whole grain flour products and concentrated sweeteners; the latter includes sweeteners, such as honey, maple syrup, molasses, cane juice, etc. The more your body is out of balance, the less tolerance your metabolism will have for eating these kinds of foods, even in small and infrequent amounts. To help you know whether something is good for you or not, think about how it was made. If it required a good deal of processing to fit it in a package, make it nonperishable, and turn it into a convenience food, it most likely is something you should avoid. Another clue is the number of ingredients. If it has more than a handful, and especially if they are hard to pronounce, you probably want to avoid it.

3. Choose lean protein the majority of the time (refer to Healthy Protein Sources on p. 20). Make sure to include protein with each meal and most snacks.

4. Eliminate manufactured fats and include healthy fats (refer to Fats That Promote Health on p. 47).

5. Eat lots of vegetables, focusing on the above-ground vegetables (see Carbohydrate Chart on p.17). Include these at least two meals out of three. Include vegetables in snacks. More is better. Root vegetables are eaten in smaller portions and less frequently, because they have more concentrated sugars.

6. Make lean protein, above-ground vegetables, and healthy fat the core of your diet. Add root vegetables, fruit, whole grains, legumes, dairy and nuts to fill out your menu. How much of these foods you add and how frequently will vary from person to person, as you will see in the sample menus.

WHAT ABOUT THE FOOD PYRAMID?

The U.S. Department of Agriculture has put forth a set of guidelines known as "the food pyramid. " The food pyramid sets the number of servings from various groupings of food that supposedly represents the healthiest diet for all Americans. Many nutritionists are beginning to question and call for a new look at the food pyramid. In light of what we know now about the importance of reducing refined carbohydrate consumption to regulate blood sugar and of the importance of healthy fats, the current pyramid is neither accurate nor adequate. And, it's simply not realistic to think that one diet could possibly take into account the varying needs and health concerns of millions of individuals. What follows are some of the considerations that will affect your dietary needs.

THE HEALING PLAN

If you need to lose more than a small amount of excess body fat, have elevated "bad" (LDL) cholesterol or triglycerides, have elevated blood-glucose levels, or are a non-insulin-dependent diabetic, in all likelihood your cells have some degree of insulin resistance and your body overproduces insulin to compensate. Your body needs a prolonged period of decreased glucose and insulin levels for your cells to become more sensitive to insulin and for your health to improve. This is accomplished by eating fewer servings per day of insulin-boosting carbohydrates. This will allow your body time to heal and possibly increase its ability to efficiently make use of carbohydrates. Many people can benefit from a period of controlled carbohydrate consumption and often find very quick relief from a variety of troubling symptoms.

If the health characteristics mentioned above apply to you, the sample Healing Menu will give you an idea of what a healthy eating style will look like. You will still be eating plenty of carbohydrates; you'll simply be choosing those that don't tax your overburdened body. As your body heals, indicated by fat and weight loss, normal blood-glucose levels, and lower bad cholesterol and triglycerides, you will gradually be able to do well with a broader range of carbohydrate choices. As an added benefit, this nutritional style will help gastric reflux, assorted joint aches and pains, fatigue, headaches, hypertension, depression, and symptoms associated with irritable bowel conditions.

73

SAMPLE HEALING MENU

BREAKFAST	LUNCH	DINNER
Omelet with sautéed mushrooms and green peppers, 1 oz. low-fat cheese ⅓ tsp. olive oil to cook Small apple or orange	Broiled salmon Tossed salad with 1 Tbsp. **Essential Herb Vinaigrette** **Steamed or parboiled broccoli**	**Chicken Fajitas** ¼ C refried beans (canned, no hydrogenated fat)
Protein Smoothie	**Gimme Five Chef Salad** 1-2 Tbsp. **Essential Vinaigrette** 1 slice 100% rye bread or 2 rye crackers	**Lemon Pepper Cod** ½ small **Baked Yam** **Steamed or parboiled * green beans**
Low-fat cottage cheese 1 Tbsp. flax meal ½ C fresh berries	**Tuna Waldorf Salad** 1 slice sprouted grain bread*	**Rocky's Mama's Turkey Meatloaf** **Cauliflower Fauxtatoes** Tossed salad
½ C Oatmeal with 1 tsp. flax oil 1 Tbsp. raisins Soft-boiled egg	**String Cheese Roll-Ups** Cherry or grape tomatoes ½ C baby carrots **Sarah's Lentil Salad**	Ground sirloin patty **Collard Greens** Tossed salad with **Essential Vinaigrette**

Bolded items appear in the Cookbook section
*Asterisked items appear in Glossary within the Cookbook

- To heal your cells from insulin resistance, give them a break from large amounts of insulin. This eating style emphasizes the above ground watery and compact (non-starchy) vegetables for carbohydrate choices. Grains, beans (legumes), fruit, and root vegetables are used less frequently and in smaller amounts. This helps keep your insulin levels low and well-regulated throughout the day. Foods from outside of the box on the carbohydrate chart (p. 17) are to be avoided. The one exception is that dried fruits may be used in *very* small quantities once in a while.

- Fats, as long as they come predominantly from olive oil, olives, nuts, nut butters, seeds, avocado, and healthy salad dressings (no sugar, corn syrup, fructose, hydrogenated fats) will not add fat to your body or increase your risk of heart disease. Of course, you cannot eat unlimited amounts, simply because too many calories in the course of the day of any kind of food will cause weight gain (unless, of course, that is your goal!) The fat to keep an eye on is the saturated fat in animal protein, such as eggs, lamb, beef, cheese, and cream. This does not mean you shouldn't have these foods; it just means the fat content of these foods should not be the major source of fat calories in your diet. You can accomplish this by choosing lean protein sources more often.

- If you are diabetic, you must be particularly careful about the use of grains, beans, fruit (including tomatoes), and root vegetables because of their potential to elevate your blood sugar out of normal range. Use your post-meal blood-sugar readings to determine if the use of foods from these categories is causing your blood sugar to elevate above 100-110mg/dl, and if it is, reduce or eliminate the offending food.

- Dairy products can be used if you are not lactose intolerant, although some people find they feel better without dairy at all. If you have frequent colds, sinus congestion, asthma, allergies, or other congestive conditions, consider eliminating dairy and seeing if it makes a difference. Skim milk should not be used because the lack of fat causes the milk sugars in it to have more of an insulin-boosting effect.

If you are not sure your health would benefit from the Healing Plan, a two-week trial will give you a sense as to whether this plan might help you.

THE MOOD-STABILIZING PLAN

If you suffer from depression, the Mood-Stabilizing Plan will help you. The brain chemistry associated with depression responds well to the ingestion of carbohydrates in small amounts throughout the day. These will help transport amino acids into your brain to be converted to the neurotransmitter serotonin.

It's also important for you to be vigilant in avoiding sugar in any form, such as alcohol and white flour products. Because of your brain chemistry, you are more vulnerable to getting caught in the downward spiral of craving foods that initially make you feel good, but leave you feeling worse and wanting more to try to feel better. Look over the sample Mood-Stabilizing Menu to get an idea of what your eating style will look like.

SAMPLE MOOD-STABILIZING MENU

BREAKFAST	LUNCH	DINNER
Scrambled eggs, **Brown Rice,** with sautéed veggies (½ C brown rice) use 1 tsp. olive oil	Broiled salmon Tossed salad 1 Tbsp. **Essential Herb Vinaigrette** Steamed or parboiled broccoli ½ C **Cinnamon Orange Squash**	**Chicken Fajitas** ⅓ C refried beans (canned, no hydrogenated fat)
Protein Smoothie 1 slice sprouted grain toast* 1 tsp. butter	**Gimme Five Chef Salad** 1-2 Tbsp. **Essential Vinaigrette** 1 slice 100% rye bread or 2-3 rye crackers	**Lemon Pepper Cod Sweet Potato Fries** Green beans with 1-2 Tbsp. chopped, toasted almonds
1 C low-fat cottage cheese 1 Tbsp. **Ground Flax Meal** ½-1 C fresh berries	**Tuna Waldorf Salad** 1 slice sprouted grain bread	**Rocky's Mama's Turkey Meatloaf** ⅓ C millet with **Tahini Sauce Collard Greens**
½ C **Oatmeal** with flaxseed oil or butter 1 Tbsp. raisins Soft-boiled egg	**String Cheese Roll-Ups** Cherry or grape tomatoes ½ C baby carrots **Sarah's Lentil Salad**	Ground sirloin patty Salad with **Essential Herb Vinaigrette** 3 oz. baked sweet potato **Steamed or parboiled Broccoli**

Bolded items appear in the Cookbook section
*Asterisked items appear in Glossary within the Cookbook

The Mood-Stabilizing Menu still uses the same core food groups as the Healing Menu. In fact, the menus are quite similar except for the addition of more servings of starchy carbohydrates like squash, whole grains, whole grain toast or crackers, and legumes. Remember that carbohydrates help shuttle amino acids into the brain to help with serotonin production. Often, people who have depression feel better simply by following the Healing Plan. However, if in following that plan your depression gets worse, you may need to slightly increase the amount of carbohydrate you eat. Notice that you still are choosing from the carbohydrate groups that fall within the box on the carbohydrate chart.

THE FIT AND HEALTHY PLAN

Are you basically healthy? I would define this as someone with all of the following characteristics:

- normal blood work (lipids, glucose, insulin, hormone levels, etc.)
- normal blood pressure
- free of sustained depression (short, situation-related depression is an occasional part of life)
- no chronic health problems
- infrequently sick from colds, viruses, etc., and if ill, recovery is not prolonged
- exercises regularly at a moderate to intense level four or more times a week
- non-smoker
- moderate or less usage of alcohol

But being healthy is so much more than the absence of illness. In addition to the above, it is, at a minimum, possessing enough vitality and energy to really enjoy your life!

I deliberately refrain from using weight or body-fat level to define health, even though it's clear that some levels of excess weight or fat are unhealthy. We have become so fixated on these as measures of health in a way that obscures a more complete picture of the person. I have never worked with a person who was significantly overweight in which there wasn't an underlying problem with metabolism related to diet and exercise habits. That may seem like an obvious statement. But, the fact is, the problems and habits of very overweight people aren't significantly different from those I see with "normal" or somewhat overweight people, with the exception of a greater genetic propensity to accumulate fat. Hypertension, high cholesterol, chronic fatigue, fibromyalgia, depression, lowered immunity, and countless other conditions of compromised health in which diet plays a significant part are equal-opportunity illnesses.

While it is true that obesity is clearly linked with many increased health risks, it is also equally true that there are health-protective effects from having a little more weight and body fat than is currently in vogue. The ultra lean look many people strive for may not be what's attainable or even healthy for you. *Your* ideal weight and body-fat level is a unique combination of your genetics, what makes you comfortable and happy, and your overall health. If you can answer yes to all of the above characteristics, and you still don't fit the "right" slot on the weight or body mass index charts, you are still a fit and healthy person. Weight or body fat loss is a matter of your personal comfort.

For the basically fit and healthy person, the Fit and Healthy Plan will keep you well-fueled. This eating style, shown in the sample menu, provides more low and moderate glycemic carbohydrates to fuel your energetic lifestyle, but still stays away from health-depleting sugars and refined carbohydrates.

The Fit and Healthy Menu still uses the same core food groups as the Healing and Mood-Stabilizing Menus. Because of the higher activity level and higher metabolism of very active people, the starchy carbohydrates like squash, whole grains, whole grain toast or crackers, and legumes can—*but don't have to be*—eaten in larger quantities. Although fruit turns to sugar more quickly than the grain and bean type of carbohydrates, people with a healthy metabolism can eat more of it. Note that carbohydrate calories still come from primarily whole, unrefined foods. As your metabolism increases, you need to consume more calories to maintain the same weight, so overall food quantity will increase.

SAMPLE FIT AND HEALTHY MENU

BREAKFAST	LUNCH	DINNER
Scrambled eggs, **Brown Rice,** with sautéed veggies (½ C brown rice) 1-2 tsp. olive oil	Broiled salmon Tossed salad with 1 Tbsp. **Essential Vinaigrette Steamed or Parboiled Broccoli** ⅔ C **Orange Cinnamon Squash**	**Chicken Fajitas,** whole wheat tortilla ½ C refried beans (canned, no hydrogenated fat) Cut-up fruit
Protein Smoothie Sprouted grain toast* 1 Tbsp. peanut butter	**Gimme Five Chef Salad** 1-2 Tbsp. **Essential Vinaigrette** 2 slices 100% rye bread or 4 rye crackers	**Lemon Pepper Cod** Small **Baked Yam** Green beans with 1-2 Tbsp. chopped, toasted almonds
Low-fat cottage cheese 1 Tbsp. ground flax meal* 1 C fresh berries	Tuna salad sandwich on 2 slices sprouted grain bread* Cut-up peppers, cherry tomatoes, baby carrots, celery	**Rocky's Mama's Turkey Meatloaf** Millet with **Tahini Sauce Collard Greens**
Oatmeal with 1 tsp. flaxseed oil or butter 1 Tbsp. raisins 2 soft-boiled eggs	**String Cheese Roll-Ups** Cherry or grape tomatoes ½ C baby carrots **Sarah's Lentil Salad**	Ground sirloin patty Tossed salad with 1 Tbsp. **Essential Vinaigrette Sweet Potato Fries**

Bolded items appear in the Cookbook section
*Asterisked items appear in Glossary within the Cookbook

DIET VERSUS LIFESTYLE

"How long do I need to follow this diet?" How long do you want to be healthy?

It is most unlikely that you never again will let sugar, white flour, or a food with trans-fatty acids cross your lips, unless you have nothing else to do with your life but focus on what you eat and you never eat away from home! What you *can* aim for is to become increasingly knowledgeable about how food affects your health and then strive to make better choices more and more of the time. As I've mentioned before, your needs will change over time, so your eating style needs to change as well.

To my knowledge, no one has methodically studied whether a metabolism that is or has become carbohydrate intolerant can reverse that damage, to what degree healing occurs, and over what time period. What I know is this:

1. Exercise plays a central role in how much carbohydrate your body can utilize. As health improves and greater levels of activity are maintained, *nonrefined* carbohydrates can be slowly increased. Each individual appears to have his or her own level of tolerance, and that may vary over time. Cues that you have exceeded your tolerance could be gaining weight, the return of symptoms that had disappeared, or feeling sluggish an hour or more after eating.

2. Refined sweeteners and refined grain products are not health-enhancing foods for anybody's diet and should not be included on a frequent or regular basis whatever your state of health.

3. Diabetics have to be more careful than most over the long term about the quantity of even lower glycemic carbohydrates. *Each incident* of elevated blood sugar poses a risk of damage to peripheral circulation, vision, kidney function, and the heart. Because these systems may already be compromised in a diabetic, the consequences of each episode of elevated blood sugar are more serious.

So many individual variables exist that while generalizations can be made, there is no single answer. One conclusion we can draw is that lack of exercise and a diet of manufactured and "predigested" foods are detrimental to everybody's health and well-being.

HOW MUCH OF WHAT DO YOU EAT?

When it comes to the term "diet," most of us are accustomed to thinking about our food in terms of a prescribed plan. That plan usually has to do with counting something (fat grams, calories, etc.) with specific limits on what we eat. This approach has some benefits and some drawbacks. The benefits come primarily from the clarity of a set program. If somebody gives you a diet to follow, you know precisely what you are to do. You can easily evaluate if you are doing it or not. The drawbacks, as I see it, are these:

- A diet often does not take individual characteristics into account.
- A diet is typically static, meaning it doesn't change as you, your body, and your circumstances change.
- A diet doesn't teach you to pay attention to your body; instead it teaches you to pay attention to the plan, which can lead you to miss vital information about your health and your diet.

For right now, I'm going to suggest that, with the exception of carbohydrates, you don't focus on the quantity of food you're eating. In working with people, my experience is that most people are not regularly overeating, although we all have occasional days of excess. More often than not, people are eating too many carbohydrates for their energy and health needs. Once the carbohydrate type and quantities are brought into balance, the rest seems to follow fairly easily. In Chapter Four, we'll talk more about adjusting your diet so your caloric intake is appropriate for your needs.

CHOOSING YOUR PLAN

If you need to, review Old Versus New Ways of Thinking, Guiding Principles and the Healing, Mood-Stabilizing, and Fit and Healthy Plans (pp. 70 -79) Decide which plan you sense best fits your needs. These plans are very similar in the types of meals you want to aim for; they vary mostly in the quantity and variety of carbohydrates recommended. So if the plan isn't the exact one for you, don't worry; you'll adjust as you go along. Here is a summary of the differences:

Healing Plan: Best for people who are insulin-resistant, diabetic, have chronic health problems, such as chronic fatigue, irritable bowel syndrome, fibromyalgia, candida (systemic yeast overgrowth), are significantly overweight, or have high "bad" cholesterol or triglycerides.

Mood-stabilizing Plan: If you suffer from depression, even if you also have any of the above conditions, you may need slightly more carbohydrates to support your brain chemistry than the Healing Plan suggests. Some people with depression do just fine on the Healing Plan and find that simply getting rid of all the processed food and sugar, and adding healthy fat, is all they need to feel better. If you follow the Healing Plan and find your depression increasing however, switch to the Mood-stabilizing Plan.

Fit and Healthy Plan: You've answered "yes" to all of the measures of health on page 77.

APPROPRIATE CARBOHYDRATE PORTIONS

In Chapter One, we discussed the glycemic index of carbohydrate food. It's cumbersome and in my opinion not very useful to memorize the glycemic index of every carbohydrate you might eat. The glycemic index may tell you something about how quickly a food turns to glucose, but its ultimate effect on your blood sugar and insulin will depend largely on how much of it you eat. I have found that my clients do well with a more practical system, first used by Dr. Barry Sears who developed the Zone Diet. Dr. Sears proposed a "block system" for measuring and evaluating carbohydrate choices. I have found the carbohydrate block to be a much more appropriate portion size than the traditional measures used by many nutritionists and health association-endorsed food plans.

A block of carbohydrate is 9 grams of carbohydrate—any carbohydrate—be it white sugar or broccoli. Nine grams of any carbohydrate will have the same effect on blood sugar with one exception. The fiber content of a food has no effect on blood sugar. Total carbohydrate grams minus the grams of fiber is called the *effective carbohydrate content*. Cooked broccoli, for example, has nine grams of carbohydrate per one-cup serving, but five of those grams are fiber. That means only four grams of the original nine will raise blood sugar and boost insulin. It would take over two cups of broccoli to raise blood sugar the same amount as 2 teaspoons of table sugar. The carbohydrate block represents a convenient portioning tool as well as a way to compare one carbohydrate to the next in terms of its effect on blood sugar, an important dimension of menu planning that has traditionally been left out of nutrition.

Regardless of calories, regardless of fat content, foods that you may have typically considered "healthy" need to be looked at through the additional lens of glucose-raising potential. When you do this, the puffed cereal with skim milk or dry bagel that you may be eating for breakfast is no longer such a great option. Foods with less impact on blood sugar leave you feeling more balanced in the hours after eating. In addition to the impact on blood sugar one would want to consider which foods would be more filling, satisfying, and nutrient-rich.

Many doctors and nutritionists who emphasize blood sugar regulation in their nutrition counseling provide a specific number of carbohydrate grams for their patients to consume; others recommend a certain number of servings (though not all use a standard serving size). I have found in practice that a range is more useful than a specific number. If I give my clients a range based on what they tell me and what I perceive their health needs to be, they can experiment and we can evaluate whether they need to adjust up or down. And that is what I propose you do as well.

Healing Plan: 45-90 grams/day divided between 3 meals and 2 snacks (5-10 blocks)

Mood-Stabilizing Plan: 90-135 grams/day divided between 3 meals and 2 snacks (10-15 blocks)

Fit and Healthy Plan: 135 grams/day divided between 3 meals and 2 snacks (15 or more blocks)

If you are more active, exercising regularly, or moving a lot in the course of your day, you will most likely use the upper end of the range.

WHAT'S IN A BLOCK

Each portion represents nine grams of *effective carbohydrate,* meaning the total amount of carbohydrate minus the grams of fiber.

Raw Vegetables

Spinach	unlimited
Lettuce	4 cups
Cabbage	3 cups
Mushrooms	3 cups
Bell Peppers	2 each
Tomatoes	2 (2½" diameter)
Mung Bean Sprouts	2 cups
Jicama	2 cups
Carrot	1 large or 1 cup sliced
Cucumber	1 each
Cherry Tomatoes	1 cup
Sauerkraut	1 cup
Snow Peas	1 cup
Onion, sliced	1 cup
Onion, chopped	¾ cup
Leeks, sliced	¾ cup
Alfalfa Sprouts	unlimited
Celery	unlimited

Cooked Vegetables (lower-glycemic)

Spinach	9 cups
Bok Choy	3 cups
Broccoli	2⅓ cups
Cauliflower	2½ cups
Asparagus	2 cups
Turnip	2 cups
Brussel Sprouts	1½ cups
Summer Squash	1½ cups
Zucchini	1½ cups
Kale	1½ cups
Collard Greens	1½ cups

String Beans	1½ cups
Eggplant	1 cup
Crushed Tomatoes	1 cup
Spaghetti Squash	1 cup
Tomato Sauce	½ cup
Pumpkin	½ cup
Lentils	¼ cup
Kidney Beans	¼ cup
Black Beans	¼ cup
Chickpeas	¼ cup
Hummus	¼ cup

Cooked Vegetables (higher glycemic)

Carrot Soup	1 cup
Puréed Squash Soup, thin	1 cup
Beets	½ cup
Carrots	½ cup
Parsnip	½ cup
Winter Squash, mashed	⅔ cup
Sweet Potato or Yam	2" x 2" piece
Baked Potato	⅓ cup
Lima Beans	¼ cup
Pinto Beans	¼ cup
Refried Beans	¼ cup
Sweet Corn	¼ cup
Peas	¼ cup
Baked Beans	⅛ cup
Tomato Paste	3 tablespoons

Fruits

Strawberries	1 cup (whole)
Raspberries	1 cup
Cantaloupe	¾ cup
Blackberries	¾ cup
Papaya	¾ cup

Blueberries	½ cup
Grapes	½ cup
Honeydew	½ cup
Pineapple	½ cup
Applesauce	⅓ cup
Apricots, fresh	2 each
Prunes, dried	2 each
Dates, dried	1½ each
Kiwi	1 each
Grapefruit	1 whole
Tangerine	1 whole
Fig, fresh	1 each
Plum	1 medium
Peach	1 medium
Cherries	9 each
Nectarine	⅔ cup
Orange	½ medium
Apple, 2¼" diameter	½ each
Pear	½ small
Banana	⅓ medium
Mango	⅓ each
Raisins	1 tablespoon
Dried Cherries	1 tablespoon

Juices

Tomato	¾ cup
Tomato-Vegetable	¾ cup
Apple Juice, unsweetened	⅓ cup
Grapefruit Juice, unsweetened	⅓ cup
Orange Juice, unsweetened	⅓ cup
Grape Juice	¼ cup
Prune Juice	3½ tablespoons

Grains and Grain Products

Popcorn, popped	2 cups
Rye Vita® Crackers	2 each

Wasa Rye® Crackers	1 each
Pancake, 4" diameter	1 each
Bagel Chip, ½ ounce	1 each
Sprouted Grain Bread, flourless	¾-1 slice
Puffed Rice Cereal	¾ cup
Corn Tortilla, 6" diameter	¾ each
Flour Tortilla, 8" diameter	½ each
English Muffin, whole wheat	½ each
Bran Muffin, 2½" diameter	½ each
English Muffin, white	⅓ each
Granola Bar	⅓ each
Hamburger Bun	⅓ each
Rolled Oats (oatmeal), cooked	⅓ each
100% Bran Cereal	⅓ cup
Bulghur, cooked	⅓ cup
Bagel, 3½" diameter	¼ cup
Pita Bread, 6" diameter	¼ cup
Pasta, cooked	¼ cup
Brown Rice, cooked	⅕ cup
White Rice, cooked	2½ tablespoons

Protein Sources that include 1 block of carbohydrate

Cottage Cheese	1 ½ cups
Ricotta Cheese, whole milk	1 cup
Ricotta Cheese, skim milk	¾ cup
Kefir	1 cup
Whole Milk	7 ounces or ⅞ cup
1% Milk	¾ cup
2% Milk	¾ cup
Skim Milk	¾ cup
Plain Yogurt	⅔ cup
Edensoy® Soymilk	⅔ cup
Tempeh	1½ ounces
30-40-40 Bar	½ each

LEARNING CARBOHYDRATE PORTIONS

To achieve the best health from your nutrition, you need to be adept at choosing high-quality carbohydrates that do not burden your body with more glucose than it can handle. The easiest way to begin is to evaluate carbohydrates for their glucose-raising potential and recognize the quantity that represents one serving. Write down some of your recent meals and figure out how many blocks of carbohydrate you eat in a typical day. For packaged foods, use the printed nutrition label to determine total carbohydrate grams minus fiber grams.

RESPECTING YOUR OWN PROCESS OF CHANGE

Okay, so now you've looked over the plans, scanned the block list, and figured out how many blocks of carbohydrate you typically eat in a day. Maybe you're freaking out a little, thinking, "I can't give up *that!*" or "So what am I going to eat for breakfast?" or "This is too hard, I can't do this." Remember: This is not a diet but a process of understanding how your body works and what it needs nutritionally so you can feel and be at your best. You will have success if you allow yourself to work on these changes over time. Most people I work with find that as they feel better from small changes, they are motivated to keep making more changes. By now, if you've been taking the steps outlined in the Nutrition Magic sections of Chapters One and Two, you probably are already noticing how much better you feel.

On the next few pages are some examples from my practice of what I mean by "respecting the process of change." I have presented the food logs from the initial consultation with four people. Each had different health needs and eating patterns and life challenges when they came in to see me. Each log is followed by how and why we determined which eating style of the three would be best for that person. Finally, you will see the recommendations I made to help the client make gradual changes to reach his or her goals. Remember, these are the *first steps* I've recommended, not the end point.

SAMPLE FOOD LOGS - LOG #1

BREAKFAST	SNACK	LUNCH	SNACK	DINNER
Tangerine 2 Doughnuts	Apple 6 pieces French bread	Spinach wrap sandwich Bag M & M's® Chocolate- covered peppermint	Snickers® bar Macaroni salad	McDonald's® fries, large Lemonade Sprite® White rice Brie cheese

Carol was severely overweight and suffered from long-standing depression, anxiety, irritability, and insomnia. She was sporadic about exercise, maintaining a program for a couple weeks that included ten to thirty minutes of an aerobic workout three to four times a week. She would also use free weights very infrequently.

Overview: Carol has a lot to change. She would benefit from the Mood-Stabilizing Plan to address her depression as well as weight. Carol's diet is filled with highly processed carbohydrates, sugar, and manufactured fats, and her eating patterns and symptoms are typical of someone with depression, highs and lows in blood sugar, and too much insulin. She is also quite resistant to the idea of giving up those foods. She grazes constantly throughout the day to offset her drops in blood sugar, and she craves food that would give her "a lift." Here are some of the things she could do to start bringing her body back into balance and reducing her cravings for sugar and refined carbohydrates.

CAROL'S FIRST STEPS
1. Start the day with some kind of protein—eggs, cottage cheese, cheese, turkey sausage. Just about anything will be an improvement and will eliminate the midmorning craving.

2. Bring a protein snack for midmorning—cheese or peanut butter to go with the apple, even cheese to go with the bread. Eventually the bread

should be eliminated, but adding cheese without taking away the bread would still help.

3. For lunch, the Spinach Wrap Sandwich isn't great because of the highly refined "wrap" and relatively low protein content, but for now a good shift might be to focus on eliminating the candy and adding a few vegetables like cucumbers and cherry tomatoes to the meal. I would also suggest a sandwich that had more protein in it and used whole grain bread instead of a refined flour-based wrap.

4. For the afternoon snack, Carol could choose more protein and some carbohydrate. If she can't get rid of the Snickers bar yet, eating part of it along with the protein would be preferable. Or switching to an energy bar of some kind (without sugar or hydrogenated fat) would be a good next step.

5. The cheese is about the only thing of value in her dinner because it provides protein, but there's too much saturated fat in that choice, given what the rest of her day looks like. I would encourage her to make sure her meal has three to four ounces of poultry, meat, or fish. Then I would suggest she work on eliminating one or two of the highly refined carbohydrate items and replace them with a serving or two of vegetables.

Comments: Adding protein will tremendously cut cravings and make other changes possible. Part of the reason change is so difficult for someone with this eating pattern is the lethargy and depression created by the diet. Protein will do a lot to give her more energy and cut her need for sugar, which in turn will help ease the depression.

SAMPLE FOOD LOGS - LOG #2

BREAKFAST	SNACK	LUNCH	SNACK	DINNER
2 cups Coffee with sugar, half-and-half 1½ Bananas ½ NutriGrain® bar		Sloppy joe on kaiser roll Extra Sloppy joe filling		Chinese "chips" Kung pao chicken White rice

Sophia had been diagnosed as hypoglycemic. She also complained of fatigue, depression, anxiety, and irritability, particularly in the late afternoons. She has a small amount of extra weight and a family history of diabetes, depression, and alcoholism. She did not feel her depression was serious enough to go on medication and had found that working out regularly helped improve her mood. She felt she was a "carboholic" because of her food cravings and was concerned that her daughter, who had been diagnosed with ADD, was eating poorly as well.

Overview: The first thing Sophia needs to address is eating more frequently to keep her blood sugar stable. Of course, the food she chooses is important too; her log shows that she at least is getting a reasonable amount of protein at two out of three meals. But her meals contain excessive refined carbohydrates and virtually no vegetables. The Mood-Stabilizing Plan would be appropriate for Sophia. She has answered "yes" to most of the questions about sugar sensitivity (p. 64). Because she is feeding her daughter too, this style of eating would meet her child's needs with only minor adjustments.

SOPHIA'S FIRST STEPS

1. Increasing her protein at breakfast would be a good first step. The 1½ bananas gives too much sugar, especially in addition to the sugar in her coffee. A protein shake with ½ small banana would be a good alternative, and cutting down to one cup of coffee would help. The coffee

provides stimulation and energy that is lacking because of the poor diet, so as more balanced meals are eaten, the need for caffeine will decrease.

2. Having snacks between meals is important for her. This would be a good place to begin adding higher quality carbohydrates. Baby carrots, cut-up peppers, cucumbers, celery with hummus, baba ghanouj, or some low-fat cheese would be quick and easy, and also a good snack for a child. Protein Nut Butter Delight (page 360) with an apple makes a great snack for adults and kids.

3. I suggested Sophia focus next on creating easy-to-prepare, balanced meals. Sloppy Joes are fine if made without sugar, and these can be made in quantity and frozen. A whole grain like brown rice or millet would be a better choice than the white bread bun. Adding a vegetable such as steamed broccoli would improve the menu, and a lot can be cooked at once and used for other meals or snacks. At a Chinese restaurant, a better choice would be a non-fried dish, preferably one with lots of vegetables. Skip the rice and fried chips. Try some Egg Drop or Hot and Sour Soup instead or a steamed spring roll.

Comments: For Sophia, ongoing changes would focus on introducing more whole grain and vegetable dishes into daily menus. This will take developing some new habits and routines for shopping and cooking so prepared food is readily available and convenient. Getting sources of healthy fat into the diet as soon as possible in the form of flaxseed oil, nuts, and nut butters is recommended and would benefit her daughter tremendously in her focus and concentration.

SAMPLE FOOD LOGS - LOG #3

BREAKFAST	SNACK	LUNCH	SNACK	DINNER
1½ cup Multigrain Cheerios® ⅓ cup 1% milk	Banana Blueberry muffin Decaf coffee	Olga® Chicken stir-fry with low-fat Olga® bread	Vanilla fat-free pudding	1 cup Black bean and rice soup ½ cup Squash ½ cup Apple sauce 1 cup No-fat egg noodles ½ cup Peas Vanilla fat-free pudding

Marlene is active and basically healthy but has a craving for sugar, which gives her headaches and makes her tired. She has gas and constipation, and would like to reduce her body fat. She has a regular exercise program of both cardiovascular and strength training. As a business owner, her life is busy and she is on the go constantly.

Overview: Marlene would benefit from the Fit and Healthy plan for eating. Her frequent consumption of large amounts of refined carbohydrates is causing her to crave sugar and more carbohydrates and contributes to her gas and constipation problems. Even with her regular exercise regimen, her body cannot burn the extra fat she would like to lose, because the high levels of insulin her diet produces lock up her fat cells. And her use of no-fat products and low-fat diet in general is working against her, making her blood sugar go even higher and slowing down her metabolism. Making time to prepare food will be her biggest challenge, but once she develops some routines, this shouldn't slow her down and will give her more energy to fuel her busy days.

MARLENE'S FIRST STEPS

1. I encouraged Marlene to first change her breakfast since it is setting her cravings in motion for the day. A protein smoothie (page 250), cottage cheese, fruit with two tablespoons ground flaxseed or a slice of sprouted grain toast with peanut butter would all be equally quick alternatives.

2. Next, she could focus on her snacks, shopping for no-preparation items: string cheese, whole grain crackers (without hydrogenated fat), fruit, prepackaged hummus or baba ghanouj. Making up Protein Nut Butter Delight (page 360) or a nut snack mix (page 193) that would last two to three weeks would be very fast. Her diet lacks vegetables and snacks would be an easy place to begin including them by washing and cutting several days' worth at once (or buying them prepared).

3 Her lunch at Olga's, without the very refined bread, would be fine; carrying her own crackers or whole grain bread would be an alternative option.

4. The dinner menu is too heavy with dense carbohydrate choices. Apple sauce could easily shift to a snack. The bean and rice soup or the squash would be fine, but not both. The noodles provide empty calories and raise blood sugar. Adding sautéed Italian turkey sausage to the soup is one example of a quick way to get more protein in that meal. Cooking a batch of turkey meatballs, boneless chicken, or a couple meatloaves would all be items that could be done in bulk and frozen.

Comments: Vegetables will be the hardest things to fit into her grab-and-go lifestyle. Steaming or parboiling a variety of vegetables once a week will give her many options for including low-glycemic vegetables in her meals. Many produce departments carry shredded cabbage, broccoli slaw, sliced mushrooms, etc., that make stir-fries very quick and able to be prepared to last for several meals.

SAMPLE FOOD LOGS - LOG #4

BREAKFAST	SNACK	LUNCH	SNACK	DINNER
Coffee with creamer Cereal Bagel with butter ·		Pasta with chicken 2 Rolls, butter Slice apple pie Coffee with creamer	Diet cola	Steak Baked potato with sour cream, butter Small salad (iceberg lettuce and tomato) Diet cola

Cliff is just moderately overweight, but his weight has been increasing gradually over the last several years. He has hypertension, elevated cholesterol, and borderline high blood sugar. He is on medication for the cholesterol and hypertension; if his blood sugar goes any higher, his doctor wants to put him on medication to regulate it. Because of his job in sales, he is on the road often and eats most of his meals out. He frequently has insomnia and lacks energy.

Overview: Cliff's symptoms and diet indicate the high probability of insulin resistance and hyperinsulinemia. It is likely that all of his symptoms can be reversed with proper diet and exercise and that he will be able, with his doctor's supervision, to taper off his current medications as his health improves. Eating on the road presents the challenge of more processed foods and manufactured fats. If he is willing to carry a small cooler with him on trips to supplement meals out, his health will benefit tremendously, but initial changes should focus on the choices he makes in restaurants to make sure he has adequate protein and a lot more low-glycemic vegetables.

CLIFF'S FIRST STEPS
1. Breakfast is the first place Cliff can make changes, going for options such as eggs or omelets and possibly some oatmeal, instead of the refined carbohydrates of cereal and bagels. These choices will keep his blood sugar and his energy levels more even all morning. Even carrying a jar of natural peanut butter to put on a bagel would be preferable to what he does now. The coffee creamer is hydrogenated and chemical-filled; milk or half-and-half would be much healthier.

2. Protein again needs to be part of lunch, but instead of pasta and rolls, a big salad and a side of a vegetable would be better. Apples carried in the car would make a good alternative to the pie.

3. Cliff's dinner is not in too bad of shape. Restaurant baked potatoes are typically huge and probably a third of one would be enough, with a teaspoon of butter and no sour cream. He could order a more nutritious salad if available, like a Caesar (hold the croutons) or a garden salad. Dressings in restaurants are typically filled with sugar and hydrogenated or manufactured oils; olive oil and vinegar would be a better choice. In addition to the salad, a double order of the vegetable of the day, light or no butter, would be a good addition. If, however, peas, corn, lima beans, carrots, or some other higher-glycemic carbohydrate is the vegetable of the day, he should skip it or order it instead of potato.

4. Caffeine, even when consumed earlier in the day, affects sleep quality as you'll learn in Chapter Five. Cliff's diet colas later in the day are probably contributing to his insomnia as well. Finding some time to get some exercise (a short evening walk or making use of the fitness facilities now in many hotels) would greatly improve his sleep, as well as his health.

5. A good strategy for people who travel a lot is to make a point of finding out where healthy restaurants are in the regions they frequent. I would suggest doing this research as an early goal for Cliff.

6. Cliff would benefit from carrying simple snacks with him in his car. This will keep him from being stranded without any good options as well as allowing him to eat snacks during the day, improving his energy and focus. Healthy snacking will also support his making better choices at mealtimes.

Comments: Thinking ahead and planning is critical for people who are on the road a lot and not in control of their food options for much of the day. Packing a cooler with healthy food, especially fresh vegetables, fruit, and protein can make a big difference. Healthy salad dressing made at home and stored in small, plastic containers could allow someone with Cliff's schedule to get some healthy fat into his diet by bringing it into restaurants for salads. Nuts, whole grain crackers, peanut butter, protein powder, and small pop-top cans of tuna fish can be kept in a container for nonperishables in the car. Low-carbohydrate energy bars are great for emergencies or to cover him during long periods of time when getting food may be impossible.

 YOUR FIRST STEPS

Review your food logs and decide on three to five steps you will take to move closer to the eating style you have chosen. Decide on the time frame for each step. Write down the steps you will take and the time period for implementing each step.

MOVING FORWARD

EXERCISE AND MOOD

Anyone who exercises regularly will tell you that part of the reason they do it is that it makes them feel great. Overweight or not, if you don't move your body, you feel sluggish and your head just isn't as clear. Exercise increases the level of endorphins in your brain and endorphins, remember, increase self-esteem and both your physical and emotional pain thresholds.

A recent study conducted at Duke University concluded that exercise was even more effective as a long-term antidepressant than medication. In this study, 150 participants (all over age 50, with a diagnosis of depression) were randomly assigned to three groups. One group took regular exercise classes, one group took the prescription drug Zoloft, and the last group used both exercise and Zoloft.

After four months, all groups showed decreased levels of depression. But after ten months, the group that was exercising only had a lower rate of relapse than either the Zoloft group or the group exercising and taking Zoloft!

Exercise is also a great stress reliever. If you're wrestling with a problem, if you're caught in thinking obsessively about a situation, taking a break to exercise can help you arrive at a solution without even trying. Stepping back from the problem, getting into your body and out of your head, seems to allow your brain and nervous system to find new pathways that can result in a "Eureka!" experience. Exercise has a demonstrated effect on blood pressure, causing hypertension to reverse and can reverse the progression of diabetes.

If you have a tendency to feel negatively about your body appearance, exercise improves your body image and your sense of yourself. The same amount of weight (whether you are "overweight" or not) feels less troublesome when your body had been energized and toned through movement. So whether it's putting on some tunes at home and dancing around your living room, walking the dog, power walking with a buddy, playing a sport, or hitting the gym, movement keeps stagnant, negative energy from accumulating in your mind!

EXERCISE AND INSULIN RESISTANCE

Insulin resistance, you remember, is the nonresponsiveness of your cells to insulin. It results from the overproduction of insulin on a long-term basis. Insulin resistance causes blood-glucose levels to remain elevated. Increased physical exercise helps your cells reverse insulin resistance when done in combination with an insulin-regulating diet. Exercise promotes muscle tissue to take in glucose, which results in lowering your blood-glucose level. Just one more reason to get moving!

 VISUALIZE YOURSELF ACTIVE!

Continue working with the visualizations and affirmations from Chapter Two, but make sure you are including, seeing, and affirming yourself being physically active and enjoying it. Remember or imagine a positive experience of moving, being athletic, flexible, graceful, or free. "Cancel" any negative thoughts or beliefs you have about not having time, being too out of shape, feeling embarrassed, being uncoordinated, etc.

GET MOVING!

Incorporate *some* activity into your life this week. Make it appropriate; you don't have to start going to the gym if you've never had an exercise routine before. Park a little further away from the store in the parking lot, walk some extra flights of stairs, go for an evening walk. There's no better time to begin than NOW!

CHAPTER FOUR

JUMPSTARTING YOUR METABOLISM

Your metabolism is the result of many chemical and physical processes that combine to sustain your physical body and, indeed, your life. In this chapter we will look at the metabolic processes resulting in excess body weight, and more specifically, excess body fat. The weight and level of fat your body maintains is referred to as its "set point." You have your very own set point determined by a combination of genetics, nutritional lifestyle, exercise habits, and a few other factors.

Our traditional notion of dieting is based on calorie reduction and ignores the fact that underneath the problem of excess fat there usually lies the problem of a metabolism too slow to process the food being eaten. I'm going to show you how your set point determines weight and fat level and how to "rehabilitate" your metabolism so it burns and utilizes food more efficiently.

In the Nutrition Magic section you will learn to calculate your appropriate calorie level and we will tackle the question of healthy, energizing breakfasts that are not carbohydrate- and sugar- laden.

In Moving Forward, you will learn about how you can use aerobic activity to "nudge" a sluggish metabolism. And we'll also consider the idea that today's cultural ideal of the lean body type is not appropriate for everyone.

UNDERSTANDING YOUR BODY

WHY DIETS ARE DOOMED

If you have ever tried weight-loss dieting, no doubt you are extremely experienced at the endeavor. Most veteran dieters know the frustration of feeling hungry, cranky, deprived, and tired. Most know the difficulty of staying with a diet over the long haul and of the anger, disappointment, and loss of self-esteem that comes with each new effort gone awry. But did you ever stop to think that maybe it was the diet that had failed you, instead of the other way around?

On the surface, the reasoning behind calorie-restrictive dieting appears to makes sense; you need to take in fewer calories than you burn to lose weight. Perhaps this idea was adapted from the experience of cultures that experienced famine. In times of famine (an "enforced" calorie restriction), people lost weight. Could it be that we re-created this "restricted access to food" scenario, hoping to mimic the results? I also can't help thinking there is a moral or punitive component to our notions of dieting. As a culture we have such a fear and loathing of body fat that we have devised all manner of denying our physical need as a form of self-flagellation.

"But wait!" you're saying. "We don't have a physical need to overeat."

True enough. We don't have a physical need to stuff ourselves beyond the point of satiation. We don't have a physiological need to eat food when we're under stress or for emotional comfort. We don't have a need to eat junk food. And all of those habits are undeniably linked for many people to their excess weight and fat. But those are not factors for everyone who is overweight or overfat, and, they are definitely not the whole story even when they are factors.

A CALORIE IS A CALORIE IS A CALORIE...NOT

Many diet "experts" are fond of saying that a calorie is a calorie is a calorie. This is often offered as a criticism of lower- or controlled-carbohydrate eating plans. According to this way of thinking, it really shouldn't matter if you eat a high-carb, low-fat diet or a low-carb, high-protein diet, or high-fat, high-water diet as long as you don't take in more calories than you expend. On the surface this makes sense; if you eat more than you need for fuel, you'll gain weight.

But it's really an oversimplification to stop here. Different kinds of calories have different effects on functions of your brain and body. Many of these have been discussed in detail already in previous chapters. If we take this fact one step further and apply it to our current discussion of metabolism, we'd find that different kinds of calories enhance or impede metabolism, particularly fat metabolism. So the same number of calories coming from different ratios of protein fats and carbohydrates will indeed have a different impact on how your body utilizes those calories. One way of eating 1500 calories may promote fat storage, while another way promotes fat-burning.

In Chapters One and Two, we discussed how the quality of the calories you eat play a significant role in what your body ultimately does with them. Eating highly processed foods, sugar, and fake or damaged fats and restricting intake of healthy fats interferes with healthy metabolism. This leads to both increased fat storage and decreased fat-burning, even during exercise.

Let's look at how your body conspires with those dietary practices to keep you struggling with weight. For some people, the most exercise they get is running on the dieting treadmill. Understanding the mechanisms that keep your metabolism from functioning optimally can allow you to get off that treadmill. Your body believes it's doing you a favor by keeping your extra pounds of fat. And you need to work with instead of against your body's innate intelligence, which is what calorie-restrictive dieting often does.

If we go back to the idea of taking in less calories than you burn and turn it around, we come up with burning more calories than you take in. Same difference? I don't think so. Most diets are designed to treat the *symptom* of a sluggish metabolism (weight and fat gain) instead of working to speed it up. This is not unlike taking a drug to cure a symptom without understanding and addressing the underlying cause of the problem. Doesn't it make sense that if the underlying problem isn't addressed, the problem will keep recurring? This is exactly what happens with the problem of fat accumulation. Diets don't address the underlying metabolic problem, so the problem keeps coming back!

Your body has a regulating mechanism in your brain that determines how much you should weigh, how big an appetite you need to maintain that weight, and how much stored fat you need in case of famine.

In these times, the conditions of famine are generally only simulated when you go on a calorie-restricted diet. Your body naturally responds to calorie restriction with a survival instinct. In other words, it says essentially, "Oh-oh, less food. Better slow things down here." Cutting calories may produce weight loss in the short term, but overall it only stimulates the body to hang on to fat and to prod you to eat more. It does this by slowing down your metabolism, increasing your appetite, and putting a stop to fat loss. And this says nothing about the sense of psychological deprivation that often accompanies unreasonable calorie restriction.

SET POINT RULES!

In a part of your brain called the hypothalamus, there is a very important cluster of cells wielding an incredible amount of power. These cells form your *weight-regulating mechanism*. This mechanism controls the level of body fat and weight you maintain, it regulates your appetite, and it controls your metabolic rate. If this mechanism were a person, millions of people who struggle with their weight would line up at the chance to dethrone this despot! The weight and body-fat level "determined" to be appropriate for your needs is called your *set point. The higher your set point, the more weight and fat you will conserve.* Your body will do whatever it can to defend its set point.

- When you go on a calorie-reducing diet, your appetite will increase to maintain your set point.

- When your body-fat level decreases, your metabolic rate slows down giving you less energy, slowing _you_ down, conserving fat, and increasing your craving for high-fat and sugary food.

- And just to make sure you don't try anything that foolish again, this autocratic collection of cells retaliates by raising your set point, causing you to eat more, burn less, and reach a higher "normal" weight.

It really does seem, sometimes, that your body is the enemy, thwarting your efforts to lose weight and get leaner. In actuality, if you understand some basics about how your weight regulating mechanism works, you can turn that despotic ruler into a cooperative ally. But you have to be willing to behave cooperatively as well.

SET POINT BASICS

If you want to work with instead of against your body, here are some things you should know about your weight-regulating mechanism:

1. Your *Basal Metabolic Rate*, also called BMR, increases when you eat more and decreases when you eat less. BMR is the amount of energy, measured in calories, that your body needs to keep you alive when at rest (i.e., doing nothing). *So eating more than your BMR increases your metabolism.* Eating less slows it down.

2. *Being physically active increases your metabolic rate*, even at times you're not being active. It's been shown that athletes have a higher BMR than nonathletes. Motion studies show that the average lean person moves more than an obese person does to complete the same task. Why? Because they have "energy to burn."

3. Your body has a special kind of fat, called *brown fat,* that is different from the white fat we'd like to get rid of. Brown fat has its own metabolic processes specifically designed to burn calories as heat, in effect wasting them to prevent them from being stored as white fat. It's been demonstrated that *lean people have brown fat that is more metabolically active* than the brown fat in the body of an obese person.

4. *Genes play a role in determining a person's set point.* Not everyone is destined to have the lean, hard-body look or the ultra-thin look that are both so trendy. There is a range of body sizes and levels of body fat that fall within the parameters of good health. While we will be discussing how to reset your set point, it's also important for you to be realistic and compassionate in your assessment of your own body. Body size and body-fat level are not the "be all and end all" measures of health.

5. Certain other factors can affect your set point. Pregnancy pushes it upward to allow a woman to conserve more stores for the growing fetus. Certain medications, notably sedatives, antidepressants and birth control

pills, also raise the set point, which is why many medications lead to weight gain. Smoking actually lowers the set point, but it does this through a very toxic and unhealthy process. This is a big reason why quitting smoking typically leads to an increase in body-fat storage. Stress can raise your set point, causing your body to hold on to or gain weight.

JUMPSTARTING YOUR METABOLISM

Even if you currently have a high set point and a sluggish metabolism, you are not doomed to live with it. You can do many things to lower it. Lowering your set point amounts to raising your BMR. If your body is able to expend more energy (calories) just to maintain basic life functions, you will create the calorie deficit needed to produce weight or fat loss without depriving your body of adequate nutrition. As we go through five strategies for raising your BMR and lowering your set point, you will notice many echo principles stated in previous chapters, reinforcing the idea that the same habits that build optimal health also support weight and fat loss.

1. If you eat fewer calories than your BMR, you will encourage your body to raise its set point and store fat. Most popular diet plans encourage a level of caloric intake that is below your BMR. In the Nutrition Magic section of this chapter, you will learn how to calculate your BMR based on your present weight and your activity level. You will see that you can still create the calorie deficit needed to lose weight without going below the BMR.

2. Physical activity on a regular basis is essential to lowering your set point. One of the primary characteristics of people who maintain a healthy percentage of body fat is that they move a lot. They get regular exercise, but they also just move more in general. They don't think twice about an extra trip up or down the stairs, for example. They move more because they have a metabolism that provides more energy, but they get more energy from moving more as well. Extended sessions (45 to 60 minutes) of aerobic activity done four to six days a week and strength training done

two to three times a week seem to be what it takes to lower a person's set point. In the Moving Forward section in this chapter and the next, we will cover the specifics you need to know to develop your own exercise program. Of course, you will start at whatever level is appropriate for you and gradually increase as you are able.

3. Avoiding sugar, refined carbohydrates, damaged fats, and excessive amounts of saturated animal fat helps to keep blood sugar, hormones, and neurochemicals balanced in the body. This balance, in turn, frees you from cravings for chemical substances, including drugs, alcohol, sugar, and refined carbohydrates, substances that keep you feeling sluggish and without energy. It also helps promote fat-burning instead of fat storage.

4. Emphasizing fiber-rich carbohydrates, especially the less-dense vegetables, along with moderate amounts of healthy fats provides a feeling of fullness and satiety that leaves you light and more energetic and improves your digestion and metabolism.

5. Eating adequate protein throughout the day is necessary to feed your lean muscle mass, which in turn stimulates fat-burning.

6. Learning to handle and release stress is an important factor in lowering your set point. Stress hormones interfere with your body's ability to metabolize fat while increasing your cravings for sugar and refined carbohydrates, the very food that leads to excessive fat storage. Exercise is an excellent way to release stress.

Putting Food and Eating in Perspective

The "dieting mentality" teaches us that less is best—eat less, think less about food. In reality, eating more food and the right kinds of food, in combination with the right kind of exercise, is what creates a fat-burning metabolism. And being more, not less, mindful of food is what allows you to plan ahead for your needs.

There is no question that it is more of a challenge, initially, to implement the dietary and lifestyle changes that lead to optimal health than it is to follow most of the diet programs out there.

Our society makes eating poorly more convenient than eating to support health. Unhealthy, manufactured food and diets form the basis for two very large industries, and junk food is available everywhere. Busy lives make taking the time to plan and prepare healthy food a low priority. Carving an extra hour out of your day to fit in exercise may seem impossible. But these are the things that it takes to have a healthy body and to feel your best— physically, mentally, and emotionally. And like any new habit, the more you do it, the more second nature it becomes. What initially may seem burdensome, what may take a lot of mental as well as physical effort over time will seem like a gift because of the rewards it brings you. The choice is yours to make.

NUTRITION MAGIC

DETERMINING YOUR CALORIE REQUIREMENTS

Use the formula on page 110 to determine your basal metabolic rate and minimum daily caloric intake.

This program is designed to free you from calorie counting. However, more often than not, people (especially those who have a history of dieting) undereat rather than overeat when they begin to pay more attention to their eating habits. This calculation will give you an objective way to evaluate how much food you need to support lowering your set point for more efficient metabolism. If you are someone who tends to overeat, having a guideline will also help you become more aware of how much food your body actually requires.

How Much Food Is Right For Me?

Below is the standard formula for figuring out your needed caloric intake based on current body weight and activity level. This formula does not take into account individual differences in metabolic rate related to age, health status, or other factors that can cause slower or faster metabolism, but it will give you a good working number with which to start.

1. Current Body Weight (BW) _____ ÷ by 2.2 = weight in kilograms(kg)____

2. BW in kg x .9 (for women only, men use BW in actual kg. number) ____

3. Number from line 2 x 24 (hours in a day) = Basal Metabolic Rate (BMR)* _____

4. BMR x Activity Factor (AF) from chart below = kcal (calories) per day to maintain weight_____

5. If weight loss is a goal, subtract 500 kcal a day from line 4 for a loss of approximately 1 pound per week_____

*Basal Metabolic Rate is the amount of energy needed for the body to perform all its involuntary functions (respiration, digestion, cell building, etc.) while at rest, but not sleeping.

Don't forget that as your weight changes or your activity level changes, your caloric requirements will change also!

Intensity	Type of Activity	Activity Factor
Very Light	Seated and standing activities, painting, driving, cooking, playing musical instrument, talking on phone, deskwork	1.3 (men) 1.3 (women)
Light	Walking 2.5-3.0 mph on flat grade, housework, waiting table, golf, sailing, ping pong, electrical trades	1.6 (men) 1.5 (women)
Moderate	Walking 3.5-4.0 mph, gardening, cycling, skiing, tennis, carrying a load, dancing	1.7 (men) 1.6 (women)
Heavy	Walking with load uphill, basketball, hockey, football, soccer, heavy digging	2.1 (men) 1.9 (women)
Exceptional	Professional athlete in training	2.4 (men) 2.2 (women)

Doing aerobic activity 3-4 hours/week = moderate
Walking or doing activities at a comfortable level without breaking a sweat = light
Not exercising = Very light

SAMPLE CALCULATION

Carla weighs 173 pounds and would like to lose 23 pounds. She walks briskly three times a week for thirty minutes each time. In selecting an activity factor for Carla, I chose the "light" AF of 1.5. Although she walks at a pace that causes her to break a sweat, the duration of her walks and the frequency, aren't enough to consider her activity level "moderate."

1. Current Body Weight (BW)_____ ÷ by 2.2 = weight in kilograms(kg)_____
   (173 ÷ 2.2) = 78.8
2. BW in kg x .9 (for women only, men use BW in actual kg. number)= _____
   (78.8 x .9) = 70.7
3. Number from line 2 x 24 (hours in a day) = Basal Metabolic Rate (BMR)_____
   (70.7 x 24) = 1697 (rounded up to next whole number)
4. BMR x Activity Factor (AF) from chart below = kcal (calories) per day to maintain weight_____
   (1697 x 1.5) = 2545 kcal
5. If weight loss is a goal, subtract 500 kcal a day from line 4 for approximately 1 pound a week loss_____
   (2545 − 500) = 2045

Carla's daily caloric need in order to lose approximately one pound a week is 2045 kcal per day.

NUTRITION-TRACKING SOFTWARE

If you would like to track how many calories you do eat, there are two simple ways to do that. One is the old-fashioned paper and pencil way. A useful book to help you with this is *The Complete Book of Food Counts* by Corinne T. Netzer.

A more exact system for keeping track of what you eat would be to use food diary/nutrition analysis software. The best, most user-friendly program I have come across is one called Lifeform. (Unfortunately, this program is not available for Mac computers.) This program allows you to log in your food, enter new recipes or frequently eaten combinations

NUTRITION-TRACKING SOFTWARE *(continued)*

into the data base, then track all kinds of health-related data if you choose, including exercise, blood-work results, symptoms, mood changes, etc. The database has the widest range of healthy foods I have come across in any nutrition software I've looked at. Best of all, it's quite inexpensive (about $40) and you can download a free trial that will last you about a month from Fitnesoft at **www.lifeform.com.** I've been using mine for several years now and I'm quite pleased with it (and I have no connection to the company!)

For Mac users, there is an inexpensive program called Cybernetic Dietician that you can download for a free trial at **www.arealinks.net/ CyberDiet.** I have no direct experience using this software.

There is other software available for personal nutrition analysis and even sites that provide free calculators for you to use. If you type "nutrition software" into any search engine on the Internet, you will find many options from which to choose. Make sure the program you use allows you to enter new foods, recipes, or meals you repeat often. Personally I look for software that has a database containing lots of fresh, unprocessed foods. (Many will consist mostly of packaged, brand-name foods and fast food items). Any software should have a free download to allow you a trial period.

THINKING OUT OF THE BOX:
BREAKFASTS FOR A REAL GOOD MORNING

After fasting all night, your brain and body both need replenishment. The typical cereal-bagel-muffin and fruit breakfast or skipping breakfast altogether sets you up for feeling tired, hungry, and mentally dull by mid-morning. A balanced breakfast supplies the energy and neurochemicals you need to be at your best and the calories needed to stimulate your metabolism into fat-burning action.

Breakfast can be challenging for people who are switching over from the typical high-carbohydrate, low-fat regime to a healthy, balanced way of eating. These next pages are designed to:

- help you shift your thinking about breakfast and breakfast food
- give you ideas and recipes for breakfasts that will keep you energized and alert through the morning
- keep your blood sugar well-regulated

First Things First

Breakfasts that include a few ounces of protein, some fat, and some complex carbohydrate (see examples below) will serve you a lot better than the typical breakfast of juice, fruit, cereal, and toast. A breakfast balanced with protein, fat, and carbohydrate will provide you with the stuff required to stay energized, alert, focused and even-tempered all morning. You might not even need caffeine to keep going! For most people who perform nonphysical types of activity, 300 to 400 calories of food will do the trick. Of course, your weight, metabolism, and energy output will determine your unique needs, but that's a rough starting point. Again, this program is not based on limiting calories, but they do give you a handy measure for making sure you are eating *enough* food.

Fruit versus Fruit Juice

I don't recommend fruit juice, since without the fiber of the whole fruit it is more highly glycemic and therefore more insulin-producing than fruit. You consume more sugar per volume drinking juice. To give you an example, you would not likely eat three or four oranges, but you consume the sugar and calories of that many in a glass of juice.

Dried Fruit

Dried fruits, such as raisins, apples, bananas, and apricots, are very concentrated in sugar. If you use them, quantities should be small (e.g., 1 tablespoon raisins, 3 to 4 apple rings) and they are best used more "condiment" style.

Are Eggs Okay for Breakfast?

For several decades, eggs have gotten a bad rap because of their cholesterol content. If you're having a conditioned-egg-avoidance response when you think about eggs for breakfast, review Chapter Two! The cholesterol in eggs will not increase your risk of heart disease if you are following a controlled carbohydrate approach. It is also fine to use a combination of whole eggs and egg whites or all whites, if you feel more comfortable doing so.

Coffee or Not?

There have been studies showing both positive and negative health effects from caffeine. Whether it's health enhancing or depleting for you will depend on your individual health status and other risk factors present in your lifestyle. Its effect also depends on the amount you drink. The truth is moderation is the best guideline if you drink coffee. Most people who drink several cups a day do so for the energy and stimulation the caffeine provides. A healthy, balanced diet will provide you with a steady energy supply throughout the day. You'll probably find you don't need a caffeine booster to get you through the day if you keep your blood sugar and insulin regulated through diet. In Chapter Five, we'll look in more detail at the potential impact of caffeine on your health.

Try Thinking Out of the (Cereal) Box!

Who says breakfast has to be limited to a particular set of foods? Any food consistent with your dietary approach that you enjoy eating is fine. Get creative! Here are some unconventional suggestions to get you started.

- Try leftover poultry, steak, other meat or fish as is, heated up, or sautéed with some vegetables.
- Toss a salad with some type of protein for a crunchy, vibrant start.
- A low-carb, creamy vegetable soup can be a soothing way to start to the day. Add a protein choice in the soup or on the side.
- Miso soup can be a nice, warming way to wake up your stomach. Make sure to include some protein, too, perhaps some scrambled eggs cooked into the soup, or some leftover chicken pieces.

- Sautéed vegetables with a small serving of leftover cooked grain (such as millet or brown and wild rice) and a couple eggs, either on the side or cooked right in after the veggies are tender, is a hearty but light breakfast. Use a little olive oil, and perhaps some wheat-free tamari (an aged soy sauce without preservatives). Make sure to stick to low-glycemic veggies like peppers, mushrooms, broccoli, bok choy, kale, collards, cauliflower, green beans, zucchini, summer squash, and red and green cabbage.

QUICK AND BALANCED BREAKFAST IDEAS

1. Omelet – 2 eggs or 1 whole egg and 2 whites, optional low-fat cheese, sautéed veggies (e.g., onions, red or green peppers, mushrooms), ½ teaspoon olive oil)

2. Omelet and baked winter squash, baked yam, or oatmeal

3. Low-fat cottage cheese and fruit, sprinkled with ground flaxseed

4. ⅔ to 1 cup oatmeal with plain whey protein powder, 1 tablespoon raisins, 1 teaspoon flaxseed oil

5. Protein smoothie with fruit and flaxseed oil

6. Soft boiled egg and chicken sausage, ⅔ cup oatmeal

7. Small piece of fruit, ½ cup low-fat plain yogurt, 2 tablespoons vanilla whey protein powder, ¼ cup granola (no sugar added variety)

8. Apple and 2 ounces low-fat cheese, 2 ounces cold chicken, 2 100% rye crackers

9. 4 ounces firm tofu scrambled with veggies, tamari soy sauce, and garlic

10. Garden burger with 1 ounce low-fat cheese, salsa (optional), small piece fruit

11. ½ cup refried beans, 2 eggs, salsa (optional)

And don't forget to look for more breakfast ideas in the recipe section at the back! Please remember to take your particular plan into account and adjust your carbohydrates accordingly.

FOCUS ON BREAKFAST

Focus on planning and eating daily, balanced breakfasts and notice the difference in how you feel. If breakfast has not been part of your routine, start with simple, light foods in small amounts, such as yogurt and fruit or a protein smoothie. If you are usually rushed in the morning, try spending a few minutes as you clean up from dinner to plan for the next morning.

MOVING FORWARD

ARE YOU HAPPY WHERE YOU'RE AT?

It's an unfortunate fact of modern life that we have become focused on weight as a measure of well-being. Although fitness is now more "in" than ever, it is often marketed as just another vehicle for attaining "the perfect body" rather than for all the ways it improves health and quality of life. The focus is now on dramatically decreasing body-fat percentage, in the same way we have focused on weight as the measure of perfection.

Don't misunderstand me. Having a healthy proportion of lean muscle to body fat *is* a valuable measure of one's well-being. It's simply that print media, the fitness and fashion industries, and Hollywood have taken even that parameter of health to the extreme. Now, instead of dieting to reach a magic number on the scale, we diet and exercise to reach a magic body fat percentage. The extremely lean physique, once the domain of professional athletes and dancers who spend their lives training and conditioning their bodies (not always healthfully) has now become the sought-after ideal for the rest of us to attain in our fifty-minute, after-work workout.

These ideals are simply not realistic for the average person juggling careers, family responsibilities, and relationships. Not every body is designed to be thin and lean, and in fact, striving for that goal can even be *unhealthy,* if your natural body type is not thin and lean. It may also take a commitment of time and energy that you don't have to attain a level of leanness that may be more than you need for good health. With all of the external messages about weight and body appearance, it can be nearly impossible to figure out what is right for you and what you truly want for yourself. Being fit and healthy, however, is realistic and attainable for most people.

Take Two Apples emphasizes attaining mental and physical health through nutrition and exercise. Everybody can benefit from that. Good food and regular exercise is the best way you have to both prevent disease and enjoy living with energy and vitality. Whether you attain a particular weight or body size is a separate question. The more overweight and out of shape you are, the less good health you are likely to possess. But it is also quite possible to be overweight by society's standards and still be very healthy and fit.

Here are some questions to ask yourself to help filter out the external noise and to focus on your unique needs and desires.

1. Do you have any conditions or a family history of conditions that put you more at risk? (diabetes, heart disease, angina, elevated LDL cholesterol or triglycerides, low HDL cholesterol, cancer, sleep apnea, arthritis, back or joint problems, stroke, hypertension, gout)
   __yes   __no

2. Do you have any chronic health conditions that interfere with your daily functioning?
   __yes   __no

3. Does your weight or body composition interfere with work, intimate relationships, social ease, or your sexual sense of self?
   __yes   __no

4. Does your weight keep you from participating in hobbies or activities that you would like to be involved in?
   __ yes   __no

5. Do you use food or weight to help you avoid dealing with emotions or situations that are difficult for you to face?
   __ yes   __no

6. Do you currently have the energy, strength, vitality, and optimism to live the life you want to be living?
   __ yes   __no

If you can truthfully answer "no" to questions one through five, and "yes" to number six, then you are probably fine, just the way you are. If you have answered that way and still don't feel okay about your weight or body, you probably have underlying issues that diet and exercise won't address. Counseling or some type of personal growth work may help you resolve these concerns.

If you answered "yes" to any question one through five, or "no" to number six, spending energy focusing on your diet and your exercise program would be a valuable investment of time and energy. And, of course, if you answered "no" to questions one through five and "yes" to number six, *and* you want to stay feeling healthy or get healthier, there is no better investment than diet and exercise.

AEROBICS FOR METABOLIC CHANGE

Having an adequately developed *aerobic system* is essential to your good health. But what exactly does this mean? Most of us have heard that aerobic exercise is any activity that gets and keeps your heart rate up. We know that brisk walking, jogging, and running are examples of this kind of exercise. But we don't usually think of ourselves as having an aerobic *system.*

The aerobic system includes your heart, lungs, blood vessels, and muscles, and it is your muscles that are the backbone of the system. It is the *activity* of the muscles that:

- increases the oxygen-carrying capacity of your blood, which feeds your tissues
- improves circulation
- strengthens your heart muscle
- increases your lung capacity
- stimulates your body's fat-burning ability

Clearly all of these functions are central to optimal health. *The majority of Americans live with health problems that are a direct consequence of an underdeveloped aerobic system.* In this chapter we'll focus primarily on improving your fat-burning metabolism because it tends to be the one symptom people worry about most. (I've never had a client come in because she feared her oxygen-carrying capacity was too low!). But excess weight and fat are only the most visible, easily identifiable symptoms of an underdeveloped aerobic system. If your aerobic system is in good shape, you will improve all the less visible but critical aspects of health as well. When fat-burning capacity increases, you not only burn visible, stored body fat, your body will also burn dietary fat before it has a chance to be stored as body fat. Your body loves to burn fat as a fuel source, but it can't do it without you activating the aerobic fibers of your muscles, which happens during aerobic exercise. A cautionary reminder, though—if you take in more dietary fat or calories in general than your body needs, you won't be burning stored fat at all, you'll be burning what you took in, and maybe not all of that!

HOW HARD DO YOU NEED TO EXERCISE?

Everyone has an ideal range of exertion or effort that will result in optimal fat-burning and conditioning of their aerobic system. I will explain below how you can determine what that range is for you. When your exercise brings your heart rate above that range, your body switches to burning primarily sugar instead of fat. You will not receive the high level of fat-burning by working at these levels, although you will still get a lot of cardiovascular and other health benefits and, if you are an athlete, performance benefits.

CALCULATE YOUR MAXIMUM AEROBIC HEART RATE

Your maximum aerobic heart rate is the maximum number of times per minute your heart can contract to pump blood. You will be exercising at a level considerably below this, but you will use this number to determine your exercise range.

1. Subtract half your age from 210. _____

2. Multiply your weight in pounds x .05 _____

3. Subtract #2 from #1 _____   Female Maximum Heart Rate

4. Men only, add 4 to # 3 _____   Male Maximum Heart Rate

Great! Now you have your maximum heart rate and you can figure out the best heart-rate range for you to accomplish your health goals.

SAMPLE CALCULATION

Carla, from our last example is 41 years old and weighs 173 pounds.

1. Subtract half your age from 210.

   (41 ÷ 2) = 20.5   (210 - 20.5) = 189.5

2. Multiply your weight in pounds x .05

   (173 x .05) = 8.65

3. Subtract answer #2 from answer #1_____   Female Maximum Heart Rate

   (189.5 – 8.65) = 180.85 (use either 180 or 181)

WHICH ZONE IS FOR YOU?

Zone One: Exercising between 50 and 60 percent of your maximum heart rate will bring you into Zone One or the *Healthy Heart Zone.* If you are new to (or returning after a long break from) aerobic exercise, this is definitely the place to start. If you are recovering from injury or surgery and healed enough to begin exercising again, Zone One is easy on your body but still effective. This is a comfortable heart rate to maintain for almost everybody and one that will result in improved blood pressure, lowered cholesterol levels, decreased stress, increased body fat utilization, and increased lean body (muscle) mass. Walking is the easiest, most accessible way to maintain the heart rate needed to be in Zone One.

Zone Two: Known as the *Temperate Zone,* Zone Two falls between 60 to 70 percent of your maximum heart rate. Exercising in this zone will give you all of the benefits of Zone One but will stimulate an even greater amount of fat burning. This is primarily because more calories per minute are burned in Zone Two than in Zone One, but the pace is still low enough that the body is pulling fat out of your fat cells to fuel your exercise. Sixty to 70 percent of your maximum heart rate can be easily maintained walking or using cardiovascular equipment, such as the treadmill, cross-trainer, Stairmaster, or stationary bicycle. Easy swimming, bicycling, or a light jog will keep you in the Temperate Zone as well.

Zone Three: The A*erobic Zone* or Zone Three ranges from 70 to 80 percent of your maximum heart rate. This is a zone for someone who has been exercising for a few months or more and is ready to work a little harder. Exercising in the Aerobic Zone produces more cardiovascular benefits than the first two zones because the heart muscle must work harder to keep your muscles supplied with blood. Your lungs are working harder to meet the increased demand for oxygen, and your body becomes more efficient at getting oxygen to all your cells. In Zone Three, your aerobic system is getting the best possible workout, *and* you are still burning fat for fuel. Although in the Aerobic Zone you are burning a lower percentage of fat—because the body is starting to utilize more carbohydrates for fuel—you are burning more calories overall to maintain this level of exercise. So, in effect, your body is burning as much fat as you burn exercising in Zones One and Two, plus you get the additional benefits of improving your cardiovascular system.

Zone Three is clearly the range in which you can get the most bang for your buck and the one you want to aim for. However, a word of caution: *Do not rush to exercise in this zone before you have built a foundation in Zones One and Two. It doesn't take too long to get here, but if you skip the groundwork, you are more likely to find yourself sore, injured, or fatigued in a way that will dampen your enthusiasm and readiness for maintaining a regular exercise program that you enjoy.*

Zone Four: This zone, called the *Threshold Zone,* is between 80 and 90 percent of your maximum heart rate. Zone Four, which improves cardiovascular strength and endurance, is a training zone for fit exercisers and athletes. In Zone Four the body burns primarily carbohydrates for fuel. If you are concerned with burning body fat, Zone Four is not the best zone for getting the job done. However, spending *some* of your exercise time in Zone

Four once you are ready to challenge yourself a little more will improve your health and sports performance.

Zone Five: Zone Five, *The Red Line Zone,* is again, a zone used by athletes in training. At 90 to 100 percent of maximum heart rate, it would only be healthy for a very fit person to periodically train in this zone. The one exception is during a medically supervised stress test during which a medical professional carefully monitors your heart during exercise on a treadmill at increasing levels of intensity.

CALCULATE YOUR IDEAL EXERCISE LEVEL

Depending on how intensely you exercise, as measured by your heart rate, you can tailor your exercise to your specific health goals. There are five heart rate ranges within which you could exercise, although we will only be concerned here with the first four. The ranges are defined by percentages of your maximum heart rate, so if you haven't completed the maximum heart rate calculation exercise above, do so now.

Zone One is **50 to 60 percent** of your maximum heart rate. Calculate that range and record it here.

_____ to _____

Zone Two is **60 to 70 percent** of your maximum heart rate. Calculate that range and record it here.

_____ to _____

Zone Three is **70 to 80 percent** of your maximum heart rate. Calculate that range and record it here.

_____ to _____

Zone Four is **80 to 90 percent** of your maximum heart rate. Calculate that range and record it here.

_____ to _____

MAINTAINING YOUR ZONE

It is important to periodically check your heart rate to see whether you are exercising at the level that will give you the benefits you desire. The most accurate way to do this is with a heart-rate monitor.

Heart-rate monitors are fastened to the chest with a band and linked to a wristwatch receiver. The chest band responds to the vibrations of the heartbeat and transmits the information to the wristwatch. They range in price from about $48 to over $200 for those used by serious, competitive athletes. The advantage of using a monitor is the constant feedback available throughout your entire exercise period without having to stop or slow down to get a reading, both of which will alter the accuracy of the reading. Many pieces of equipment in gyms today have built-in heart-rate monitors.

But it certainly isn't necessary to invest in a heart-rate monitor to get the benefits of aerobic exercise. Millions of people exercise without one and are getting aerobically fit. If you don't use a monitor, you should check your pulse—either on the inside of the thumb side of your wrist or just in front of the carotid artery on your neck—periodically during exercise. Try to find the pulse as quickly as possible, since a delay of even a few seconds will give you a less accurate reading. Take a six-second count, which should be equal to one-tenth of your target rate. Eventually, you will get a good sense of what exercising at your target rate feels like.

TAKING YOUR PULSE MANUALLY

In either place, find your pulse immediately after stopping exercise. Take a six-second count and multiply by 10.

Radial Pulse: Take two fingers, preferably the 2nd and 3rd finger, and place them in the groove in the wrist that lies beneath the thumb. Move your fingers back and forth gently until you can feel a slight pulsation. Don't press too hard, or you'll just feel the blood flow in your fingers.

Carotid Pulse: The carotid arteries supply blood to the head and neck. Find this pulse by taking the same two fingers and running them alongside the outer edge of your trachea (windpipe). This pulse may be easier to find than the radial pulse. Use only very light pressure or your will get an artificially low reading.

CHALLENGING YOURSELF

As your fitness level increases, you will need to work harder to reach your target rate, another reason why monitoring in some way is important. These increases signal progress! If you are overweight you may have been told that you should exercise at a lower level to burn more fat. But remember, as your aerobic system becomes more fit, you will need to increase your workout intensity to continue burning fat. The more fit you are, the more you can consistently work out in Zone Three, with intermittent periods in Zone Two and Zone Four during your workouts. If you find yourself reaching a plateau in weight or fat loss after you have been consistently exercising and have developed a base level of fitness, it may well be a sign that your body is ready to work a little harder.

SMART HABITS FOR THE LONG TERM

Duration and Frequency: In order to lower your set point, you want to work up to exercising for forty-five to sixty minutes, five to six days a week. If you are just starting to exercise, twenty minutes is sufficient, or if you can't do twenty minutes, do what you can. Maintain a certain level for at least three weeks, then increase by five- to ten-minute intervals, maintaining each for a few weeks as well.

Types of Exercise: Any exercise that you will do, that you like, and that will maintain your target aerobic heart rate is good for lowering your set point. Walking is often the easiest and most pleasant for people to do. It requires no special equipment or facilities and it's usually easy to find a buddy or two to go with you. You can also use the time to either listen to audiotapes, music, or simply to relax and enjoy a meditative time to yourself. Biking, swimming, easy jogging (if you have no knee, back, or joint problems), or using a stationary bike, treadmill, or cross-trainer at the gym are also effective. If you have much extra weight, jogging is too stressful on your body and doesn't provide any benefits you won't also get by walking. Having two or three different things you like to do will provide extra benefits, since no two exercises use exactly the same muscle groups. Plus, you'll get variety, which will keep you from feeling bored.

Warming Up, Cooling Down: Warm-up is the ten- to fifteen-minute period during which you gradually take your activity level up to your target heart zone. This time warms up your joints and muscles, including your heart muscle, by slowly increasing blood flow. It also allows your muscles to begin breaking down fat to provide fuel for your activity. (However, remember that your body cannot access fat for fuel if insulin is present.) After you have exercised at your target heart rate for a period of time (ideally a minimum of thirty minutes), allow your body to cool down and your heart rate to return to normal by doing your activity at a steadily decreasing pace for ten to fifteen minutes. Both of these pre and post periods are important to preventing injury and getting the most from your exercise. Performing some light stretches after you exercise, when the muscles are still warm and pliable, will help increase your flexibility and decrease any soreness you might feel from the exertion.

Water and Hydration: Keeping your body well-hydrated with plain water while you exercise is essential. Get in the habit of carrying a water bottle with you. If you walk, a waist sack that holds a water bottle allows you to keep your hands free. Look for one that centers the water bottle on your lower back so you don't have an uneven weight on one side of your body. Even if your activity is swimming, you need to drink water during your workout. Just because you're *in* water, doesn't mean your body is being hydrated (unless—and let's hope this isn't the case—you're swallowing a lot of the water)!

Staying With It: When you have an underused aerobic system, exercise and staying with it beyond a few weeks is often difficult. If your set point is high and you're carrying extra body fat, your body wants to conserve energy, and it does this by slowing you down. Getting moving and staying moving may feel like it goes against your natural impulse and it may be hard for you to stick with your intention to exercise regularly. I encourage you not to give in to this inertia if it hits you. By anticipating this possibility, you can use your intelligence and good planning to outwit that sly trickster, your set point! Here are some possible strategies:

- Make a commitment to someone else to exercise together.
- Keep your exercise at a regular time, built into your schedule.
- Incorporate something you need to get done into your exercise (walking a dog, doing an errand).
- Reward yourself with something other than food for "a good record".
- Every few weeks, try on an article of clothing you want to fit into to gauge your progress.
- Visualize yourself being active and enjoying it.
- PLAN to succeed!

You *will* reach a point where being active feels better than being inactive. This is a real milestone, when you no longer have to worry that, if you miss a few days of exercise because of some extenuating circumstance, you'll fall back into your couch-potato ways. Your body will give you the clear message that you want to move because you feel good when you do. In the meantime, use your visualizations and affirmations to strengthen an internal sense of yourself as moving effortlessly and with pleasure.

If you are truly ill or injured, however, take a break from exercising to allow your body the time it needs to heal. Then, start off with shorter periods of time and, if needed, less intensity than before you stopped, and build up as you can.

SOMETIMES LESS IS MORE

I know, from personal experience, that it is easy to push yourself to exercise harder, believing more is better; this is certainly a cultural attitude that many of us have adopted. But often, less is more. If you have been exercising at the aerobic level or above and are not getting the fat-loss results you want, or if you have nagging aches and pains, try dropping down to Zone Two for a while. You will most likely find that your body appreciates the rest and will reward you with the results you're looking for.

PLANNING FOR AEROBIC HEALTH

Make a plan for tuning up your aerobic system and lowering your set point.

- What activity or activities will you do?
- Do you want to include a buddy? Who? When will you contact her or him?
- What day will you start?
- How much time will you exercise to start, including warm-up and cool-down?
- When will you fit the activity into your schedule?
- What is your target aerobic heart rate?
- Practice taking a measure of your heart rate if you have not done this before.
- Get a water bottle if you do not have one.

CHAPTER FIVE

SOMETHING TO DRINK— MORE THAN AN AFTERTHOUGHT

How much thought do you give to the health effects of what you drink with or between your meals? Is caffeine a regular part of your daily diet? What about soft drinks? Do you pay attention to how much water you drink, and do you try to drink eight to ten glasses a day all year round? What you drink or don't drink can be as important to your physical and emotional health as the food you eat, yet beverages usually don't get much attention from either individuals or health professionals. This is unfortunate since coffee and soft drinks are virtually the national beverages, and both can have a serious negative impact on health.

While most Americans are aware of the importance of drinking water on a daily basis, only about a third follow this recommendation. Dehydration is one of the most common and easily reversible contributing factors to fatigue, high cholesterol, hypertension, skin problems, fibromyalgia, joint aches and pains, weight gain, headaches, gastrointestinal problems, and other disease conditions.

In this chapter, we will look at some of the health consequences of what you drink and don't drink and discuss strategies for developing healthier habits. The Nutrition Magic section will show you how to wean yourself off caffeine without the agony of the caffeine headache. Often coffee, tea, and soft drinks become a part of your routine to compensate for inadequate sleep, so in Moving Forward we'll discuss the issue of sleep and look at ways you can improve yours.

UNDERSTANDING YOUR BODY

The short of it is, caffeine is an addictive drug with serious negative health consequences. Yet it's a drug we not only legalize, but readily promote as part of social ritual. I suspect if the average person and the average health professional took the time to understand how caffeine affects both body and mind, we would reconsider our behavior.

Coffee is the second most highly traded commodity in the world, the first being petroleum. Perhaps that's not so surprising, considering most people use coffee to "fuel" their energy.

The average per capita consumption, worldwide, is estimated to be 200mg per day, including coffee, tea, soft drinks, and chocolate. But in reality, among caffeine users, a typical day's consumption is much higher, because "average per capita" consumption is calculated by dividing the total amount of caffeine produced by the total world population. Obviously, not every man, woman, and child consumes chocolate, soft drinks, tea, or coffee, and among those who do, individual consumption varies considerably. And the many over-the-counter and prescription drugs containing caffeine are not even included in this figure. In any case, what's really important is *your* consumption, not the average. You'll have a chance later to evaluate your own caffeine consumption and decide if you're putting your health at a disadvantage.

Caffeine use by children and teenagers, mostly through the consumption of soft drinks, is a growing health concern. On top of that, the sugar added to their diets from soft drinks (averaging 9 teaspoons per 12-ounce can) is a major contributing factor to weight problems and the epidemic of "adult" onset diabetes that is affecting children in the United States.

Coffee, the primary source of caffeine for most people, is a health hazard not just because of the effects of caffeine and other chemicals naturally contained in coffee, but also because of the toxic man-made chemicals that are used in its growing and processing. Coffee plantations are heavily sprayed with pesticides to control insect infestations. Decaffeinated coffee, unless it is decaffeinated using a chemical-free, water-processing method, contains even more toxins, because chemical solvents are used to extract the caffeine.

THE EFFECTS OF CAFFEINE ON THE BODY		
Nervousness	Upset stomach	Gastrointestinal irritation
Headaches	Hypertension	Increased risk of stroke
Anxiety	Heartburn	Increased risk of heart disease
Irritability	Ulcers	Blood sugar elevation
Agitation	Diarrhea	Heart arrhythmia
Insomnia	Fatigue	Nutritional deficiency
Tremors	Poor concentration	Decreased immunity
Depression	Mood changes	Fetal growth retardation

ENERGY, BUT AT WHAT COST?

You may enjoy the taste of coffee, but you probably enjoy the taste of lots of things that you don't consume every day. If you are a regular coffee drinker or you drink caffeinated soft drinks regularly, do you use them for the lift they seem to give you? Do you feel groggy and lethargic in the morning until you've had your "morning cup" or do you "cure" your afternoon fatigue with a caffeine-containing soft drink? Would it be hard for you to give up coffee or caffeine-containing soft drinks because of the stimulant effect they provide?

Although caffeine temporarily provides a boost in energy, it actually contributes significantly to fatigue; but since the resulting fatigue occurs over the long run, it is not associated with the caffeine. Caffeine causes fatigue, by putting the body in a highly stressed state, stimulating the adrenal glands to produce epinephrine and norepinephrine, the hormones that trigger our "fight or flight" response. In this state of emergency, heart rate increases, blood pressure goes up, and a cascade of other events are initiated. General constriction of blood vessels occurs, reducing oxygen flow to the brain and all tissues. It is this vasoconstriction that leads to elevated blood pressure. Even a moderate amount of caffeine in a healthy individual can produce borderline hypertension. You feel more alert on caffeine, but only because you have put your body in a state of hypervigilance. This state of emergency, imposed day after day on your organs and body systems, is very depleting to your health and well-being.

When the body's fight or flight mechanism is triggered, the liver puts more glucose into the blood to provide the energy for fight or flight. This is a primitive survival mechanism no longer appropriate for most daily situations we face. Although it may sometimes feel as though your work or your kids pose a threat to your sanity, these are not typically situations for which you need this basic instinct! So elevated blood sugar (and its partner, increased insulin) in this case, potentially poses other problems for your body, as you certainly know from previous chapters.

STRESS HORMONES WREAK HAVOC

Caffeine also stimulates the adrenal glands to produce the stress hormone cortisol. If you remember from Chapter Four, "Jumpstarting Your Metabolism," stress hormones inhibit your body's ability to burn fat, leading to excess fat storage. So the idea of caffeine-containing drinks being an aid to weight loss is not actually true. While caffeine may depress appetite, remember that the combination of eating fewer calories than your body requires to sustain basic functions (your basal metabolic rate) and producing more stress hormone will actually lead to a raising of your set point and, ultimately, to weight gain. And you may find, that if you use caffeine for its appetite suppressing effects, you do a lot of "rebound eating" at the end of the day when the effects have worn off and your body is clamoring to be fed. Eating more at the end of the day, when you are less active and your metabolism naturally slows down, will lead to weight gain and fat storage.

The increased cortisol production also interferes with the secretion of melatonin, a hormone important both to sleep and immunity. Melatonin regulates your sleep cycles, and without adequate amounts of it your body has difficulty achieving the deepest stage of the sleep cycle, the most restorative and healing part of sleep. So even if caffeine is stopped early enough in the day to prevent keeping you awake at night, it may be lessening the quality of your sleep and increasing your level of fatigue.

Melatonin is also a major antioxidant that helps restore your immune system every night as you sleep. This suppressed production of melatonin compromises your immunity. Caffeine reduces the activity of monocytes and NK cells (natural killer), two types of cells that are an important part of your immune system.

Under various types of psychological or social stress (in other words, when you're uptight), your body's stress hormones are called into action. *Caffeine more than doubles this response!* Regular consumers of caffeine are more likely to experience irritability, tension, depression, anxiety, or panic than are nonusers.

There's another very important link between caffeine, stress hormones, and your health. When your adrenal glands are forced to work constantly, they begin to wear down. This is called *adrenal exhaustion* and one of its key symptoms is that you feel exhausted. Your body is unable to recover a sense of vitality and energy, even after a good night's sleep. Adrenal exhaustion is often an underlying piece of chronic fatigue, fibromyalgia, and other autoimmune diseases. When the adrenals are exhausted, they are no longer able to produce sufficient cortisol when the body does need it, such as in response to inflammation or allergies. Remember that cortisol is your body's natural anti-inflammatory.

NUTRIENT DEPLETION

Caffeine is known to interfere with several mechanisms of the gastrointestinal tract involved in digestion, absorption, and elimination of the food you eat. It causes irritation of the lining of your gastrointestinal tract, which in turn can lead to symptoms of irritable bowel syndrome as well as poor nutrient absorption. Studies also show that B vitamins are lost through urine when caffeine is consumed and the absorption of important minerals, such as calcium, iron, magnesium, potassium, and zinc, is reduced.

Women need to know that caffeine use can increase their likelihood of anemia (low iron levels) because of its interference with iron absorption. Women who menstruate usually have low iron levels due to monthly blood loss, so they are especially vulnerable to this iron-depleting effect. Older women need to be concerned with the impact of caffeine on bone density because of the way caffeine interferes with calcium absorption.

GENDER INEQUALITY

Like many other aspects of society, when it comes to caffeine, women are not treated the same as men. As with most drugs, women have a stronger reaction to a given dose than men do. In part, this is due to the fact that many women have a lower body weight than an average man. But the half-life of caffeine in women, that is, the time it takes for 50% of the drug to leave a woman's body, is longer than it is for men. And the half-life increases additionally in the second half of the menstrual cycle (the two weeks prior to a period). In women who use oral contraceptives, the liver becomes less effective in detoxifying the body from caffeine and the half-life doubles.

Caffeine use has been linked with delayed conception, and sudden infant death syndrome and is a known causal factor in fetal growth retardation.

THE HEART DISEASE CONNECTION

In the late nineties, a new risk factor came to our attention as a leading predictor of heart disease: the biochemical *homocysteine*, a by-product of meat and dairy proteins. When health is good, homocysteine is normally broken down and eliminated from the body. However, when this doesn't happen and homocysteine accumulates, it is damaging in several ways directly related to heart disease. And caffeine consumption and elevated homocysteine levels are also directly related; that is, the more caffeine you consume, the higher your homocysteine level.

Research suggests, homocysteine causes damage to blood vessel walls. When blood vessel walls are damaged, protein, calcium, and cholesterol are deposited in the damaged areas to try to repair the walls. This patching material, made from cholesterol, is what you may know as plaque. Although it is a very necessary material, plaque build-up leads to narrowing of the arteries. So the more caffeine you consume and the higher your homocysteine levels, the more at risk you are for blocked arteries as your body keeps adding plaque.

Homocysteine also cause blood platelets to become stickier, which increases the likelihood of blood clots to occur. Increased blood clotting is more likely to lead to stroke, especially if the arteries are narrowed to begin with from plaque build-up. Homocysteine has also been shown to impair the elasticity of blood vessels, which in turn reduces their ability to expand. If your arteries cannot expand each time your heart pumps more blood through them, your blood pressure increases.

Every risk factor for heart disease is compounded by caffeine consumption. A study published in 1997 in the *Journal of the American Heart Association* concluded that people with highest homocysteine levels had over three times the risk of heart disease as those with low homocysteine levels. Caffeine is thought to raise homocysteine levels in two ways: One is that it simply interferes with the breakdown process; the second is that it depletes the body of the B vitamins that are essential to the elimination of homocysteine from the body.

CAFFEINE AND BLOOD PRESSURE ELEVATION

Caffeine causes an elevation in blood pressure because it causes more constriction of blood vessels. If you already have hypertension, you especially want to examine your caffeine use.

When you exercise, your blood pressure naturally elevates due to the increased demand for blood flow. If you use caffeine throughout the day or have several cups of coffee or a large amount of a caffeinated soft drink before you work out, you will be compounding the blood pressure increase.

THE CAFFEINE BRAIN DRAIN

Think coffee makes your thinking sharp? Think again! The constriction of blood vessels from caffeine affects blood vessels in your brain. In fact, only 250mg of caffeine can decrease blood flow to the brain as much as 30 percent! One 16-ounce mug of coffee (travel mug size) can deliver that much caffeine to your system. If your brain gets less blood, which is the delivery vehicle for oxygen and nutrients, how can you possibly be as mentally sharp with caffeine as you are without it?

SOFT DRINKS: HARD ON YOUR BODY

Industry-gathered data shows that as of 1995, the average soft drink consumption in the U.S. was equivalent to 546 12-ounce servings per person per year or just under 1½ ounces per day. Since not every man, woman, and child consumes them, many of us are drinking a great deal more than that. In the 1950s, Coca-Cola®, the leading soft drink at the time, came in 6-ounce bottles; now a single serving of all soft drinks is likely to be 12, 20, or even 64 ounces!

Many of these drinks contain caffeine, and not just the colas, as you might expect. Mountain Dew®, Sunkist Orange Soda®, and Dr. Pepper® all contain caffeine and in some cases contain *more* of it than the leading cola brands. Caffeine-containing soft drinks are growing annually in sales.

In addition to the caffeine content, soft drinks present several other negative health consequences. The most obvious is the sugar content; the average 12-ounce soft drink has 3 tablespoons of sugar in it. Drink a 20-

ounce bottle and you've consumed almost a ⅓ cup of sugar! Think of the impact on blood sugar of drinking one or more of these every day or, as some people do, drinking one or more "super-size" soft drinks of 64 ounces each!

The sugar-free varieties are sweetened with chemical sweeteners that have been linked with behavioral and neurological problems, despite the FDA claims that artificial sweeteners are safe. Phenylalanine, one of the components of artificial sweeteners, is an amino acid that competes for absorption in the brain with tryptophan. You'll remember from Chapter Three, "Good Meals, Good Mood," that tryptophan is the amino acid that converts to serotonin, a neurotransmitter essential in combatting depression. While artificial sweeteners have not yet been linked expressly with depression, studies have linked depleted tryptophan levels with amino acids that compete with it, such as phenylalanine. So it isn't too far of a leap to associate artificially sweetened soft drinks and other chemically sweetened food and beverages with depression, especially with high levels of consumption of these products.

Bones don't like soft drinks, either. Soft drinks contain phosphoric acid, a form of phosphorus, which binds with calcium and prevents it from being used to strengthen your bones. More calcium than the amount "stolen" by phosphorus would have to be ingested to compensate. But most people don't take in enough calcium to begin with, and children especially, are drinking less milk, their chief source of calcium, in favor of soft drinks. On top of that, both sugar and caffeine lead to poor calcium absorption and calcium loss, depleting the body even further. For women, who need to protect their bone mass for later years, and children, who are still accumulating bone mass, regular consumption of soft drinks is a major assault on bone density.

HOW MUCH IS TOO MUCH?

Most studies that suggest a connection between negative health effects and caffeine show effects at upwards of 200mg per day. The more compromised your state of health, the more likely it is that you will suffer negative consequences at lower doses. And remember, the majority of studies have been done on men; women react more strongly at lower doses.

WATERING THE GARDEN OF HEALTH

Your body is composed of 75% water, and your brain, 85%. It's amazing that the largest constituent in the body is given such little recognition. Our current model of understanding the human body gives water a back seat to all the solid parts of our structure. Does it make sense, though, that all that water is there merely as filler or as a transporting agent for the "real" stuff of life?

In *Your Body's Many Cries for Water*, Dr. F. Batmanghelidj offers a compelling biological discussion of the role of dehydration in illness. Many illnesses, according to Dr. Batmanghelidj, are signals or symptoms of dehydration. When we use medication to treat these symptoms, we are ignoring the underlying cause—lack of sufficient water—allowing the illness to progress.

Batmanghelidj explains that as we evolved from sea-dwelling amphibians to land-dwelling mammals who ventured further away from water, we had to develop survival mechanisms to compensate for times of water insufficiency. The body is designed to conserve water when necessary and route it to the most essential organs. This results in parts of the body going without adequate water in order to spare more critical organs and functions. Our bodies give various pain and dis-ease signals when we are dehydrated—headaches, joint pain, fatigue are common. Thirst, the signal we are most familiar with, occurs only when the body is already dehydrated!

Lack of sufficient water can affect every system of your body, because every part of your body depends on water as a carrier for substances such as sodium and potassium. But water serves a more important role than merely transporting these minerals. Our bodies need to have a precise balance of water on the inside and the outside of cells to make sure our "chemical soup" has the right concentration. When it doesn't, your body can't function properly, and it creates various biochemical reactions to compensate for the lack of water balance. We rarely connect symptoms such as headache, fatigue, muscle and joint pain, or ulcers to something as simple as inadequate water, but these things often reverse themselves or lessen when enough water is consumed. I had one client with fibromyalgia who started drinking more water every day and found her pain diminished considerably from this single intervention. In my own experience, and those of many clients, drinking more water has alleviated headaches, joint pains, gastric disturbances, and dry skin conditions and improved athletic performance and exercise recovery. What a simple, low-tech, low-cost solution!

Most health information tells us that dehydration can occur as a result of bleeding, diarrhea, vomiting, sun and heat exposure, or certain medications. Interestingly, our failure to drink water is rarely identified as a cause of dehydration, yet it is probably the most common cause!

CHOOSING WHAT TO DRINK

The excessive use of coffee, tea, and soft drinks is linked to dehydration in two ways. First, many people choose soft drinks or coffee over plain water when choosing what to drink. Children are not taught to drink water. We are conditioned and have conditioned our children to think we must have "tasty" beverages. Second, these beverages often contain ingredients that additionally cause water loss to the body through their diuretic action, meaning they actually cause water loss.

Ideally, we should consume 1/2 ounce of water per pound of body weight every day, and more during exercise or physical activity. Water not only hydrates the body, but also keeps us healthy by flushing out toxins as the body detoxifies. Detoxification occurs constantly in the healthy body, as our bodies get rid of poisons that we may take in through pollution, pesticides, medications, chemical contaminants in food, or toxic by-products of our metabolism. A build-up of toxins is frequently connected to poor health, as the body simply cannot function as well when it is filled with toxic waste. Drinking filtered water from which chemical or bacterial impurities have been removed is important to good health.

NUTRITION MAGIC

CAFFEINE USE AND IMPACT ASSESSMENT

You may already know in your gut that your caffeine use is excessive or that it interferes with your health and well-being. Or maybe you're not sure whether you take in enough caffeine on a daily basis to worry about it. The following exercise will help you look objectively at how much you take in. Then you can decide, based on those results and on everything you've read in this chapter, whether you want to work on decreasing your consumption.

Using the "Caffeine Content of Food and Drugs" list that follows, make an assessment of your daily caffeine intake. Then answer the questions on page 143.

CAFFEINE CONTENT OF FOODS, BEVERAGES, AND DRUGS	Serving size	Caffeine in mg	For each additional ounce add
COFFEE (Coffee strength varies widely; these are average numbers)			
Drip	8 oz	216	27
Percolated	8 oz	182	23
Instant	8 oz	92	12
Decaffeinated	8 oz	6	.7
TEA			
Black Tea, brewed one minute	8 oz	43	5.4
Black Tea, brewed three minutes	8 oz	65	8
Black Tea, brewed five minutes	8 oz	71	9
Canned Iced Tea	12 oz	70	6
Green Tea	8 oz	30	4
Celestial Seasonings® Herbal Tea	Any	0	0
Snapple® Green Tea with Lemon	16 oz	32	2
Snapple Lemon Tea, Diet or Regular	16 oz	42	2.6
Snapple Mint Tea	16 oz	42	2.6
Snapple Peach Tea	16 oz	42	2.6
Snapple Raspberry Tea	16 oz	42	2.6
Snapple Diet Raspberry Tea	16 oz	42	2.6
Snapple Sun Tea	16 oz	10	.6
SOFT DRINKS			
Coca-Cola®	12 oz	34	3
Diet Coke	12 oz	65	5.4
Mellow Yellow®	12 oz	51	4
Tab®	12 oz	47	4
Dr. Pepper, Diet Dr. Pepper®	12 oz	41	3.4
IBC® Cherry Cola	12 oz	23	2
Ruby Red Squirt®	12 oz	39	3
Sunkist Orange®	12 oz	41	3.4
Sun Drop®	12 oz	63	5
Diet Sun Drop	12 oz	69	5.7
Mountain Dew, Diet Mountain Dew®	12 oz	55	4.6
Pepsi Cola®	12 oz	38	3
Diet Pepsi	12 oz	36	3
Pepsi One	12 oz	55	4.6
Wild Cherry Pepsi	12 oz	38	3

CAFFEINE CONTENT OF FOODS, BEVERAGES, AND DRUGS	Serving size	Caffeine in mg	For each additional ounce add
Royal Crown Cola®	12 oz	43	3.6
Jolt®	12 oz	71	6
Ginger Ale®	12 oz	0	0
Root Beer	12 oz	0	0
Minute Maid® Orange Soda	12 oz	0	0
CHOCOLATE			
Baking Chocolate	1 oz	35	35
Bittersweet	1 oz	25	25
Semi-sweet	1 oz	20	20
Milk Chocolate	1 oz	6	6
Cocoa (mixed, hot)	8 oz	14	1.8
YOGURT			
Dannon® Coffee Yogurt	8 oz	45	5.6
Yoplait® Café Au Lait	6 oz	5	1.2
Stoneyfield Farm® Cappuccino Yogurt	8 oz	0	0
ICE CREAM, FROZEN YOGURT			
Ben and Jerry's® No-Fat Coffee Fudge Frozen Yogurt	1 cup	85	
Starbucks® Coffee Ice Cream, assorted flavors	1 cup	50 (avg.)	6.2
Häagen Dazs® Coffee Ice Cream	1 cup	58	7.3
Häagen Dazs® Fat-Free Coffee Frozen Yogurt	1 cup	40	5
Häagen Dazs® Low-Fat Coffee Fudge Ice Cream	1 cup	30	3.8
Starbucks® Frappuccino Bar	1 each	15	
Healthy Choice® Cappuccino Chocolate Chunk, Cappuccino Mocha Fudge Ice Cream	1 cup	8	1
MEDICATION			
Caffedrine® Capsules, No-Doz®, Vivarin®	1 each	200	
Pre-Mens Forte®, Permathene Water Off®	1 dose	200	
Anacin®, Midol®	1 tablet	64	
Bufferin®, Aspirin®, Tylenol®	1 tablet	0	
Excedrin®	1 tablet	130	
Vanquish®	1 tablet	66	

1. Including coffee, tea, soft drinks, chocolate, and medication, how much caffeine are you getting on a daily basis?

2. Do you have any problems with sleep quality or quantity (i.e., do you feel rested and refreshed when you wake up in the morning?

3. Do you experience a high amount of stress at work or at home?

4. Do you have high blood pressure?

5. Do you have heart problems or a family history of heart disease or problems?

6. Do you smoke?

7. Do you or does anyone in your family have diabetes?

8. Are you significantly overweight?

9. Do you find yourself out of breath when you walk up stairs or do other lightly exerting tasks?

The more "yes" answers you have on questions 2 through 9, the more likely it is that caffeine is adding to your risk factors for heart disease, stroke, hypertension, fatigue, and complications of diabetes.

If you have an autoimmune disease, such as chronic fatigue, fibromyalgia, rheumatoid arthritis, or lupus, or if you have fibrocystic breasts, you would do best to avoid caffeine altogether to assist in healing your body. If you have hypertension, diabetes, and heart disease or have had a stroke, caffeine clearly increases your risk for all of these. The more you consume, the more you are increasing your risk.

CAFFEINE DETOXIFICATION

You are the only one who can determine if you need to scale back or eliminate caffeine from your diet. If you have decided that it's time to do that, the "Caffeine Detoxification Guidelines" will help you wean yourself off caffeine in a way that will minimize any uncomfortable withdrawal symptoms.

One of the biggest roadblocks to people reducing or eliminating caffeine from their diets is the occurrence of the "caffeine headache." Caffeine withdrawal is very real and needs to be taken seriously. While not life-threatening, the symptoms are quite uncomfortable and can sabotage your efforts to change your habits. In addition to the pounding headache that typically accompanies caffeine withdrawal, being more tired, cranky, and on edge are often parts of the withdrawal.

AVOIDING THE HEADACHE

The caffeine headache is a result of blood vessels quickly expanding. Remember that one of the effects of caffeine is vasoconstriction or constriction of blood vessels. This constriction reduces blood flow. When blood levels of caffeine drop suddenly, as they would if you stopped cold turkey, blood flow to the brain is suddenly increased and results in the infamous headache. To avoid this, a slow and steady reduction in the amount of caffeine over a several-week period should be used. Remember that coffee, chocolate, tea, and caffeinated soft drinks all need to be taken into consideration if they are a regular part of your diet. If you regularly use caffeine-containing medication, or you take any medication that you suspect may have caffeine, you may want to discuss this with your physician.

CAFFEINE DETOXIFICATION GUIDELINES

There are several strategies you can use. Let's focus first on coffee drinkers.

1. Gradually reduce the size of the coffee cup you're using. Most mugs today are 12 or 16 ounces compared to the 8-ounce coffee cup so common twenty years ago. Don't fill your mug as full or get a smaller one.

2. Slowly introduce either decaf coffee (water-processed only) or an herbal or grain coffee (see below) into your mixture so you are gradually decreasing

144

the proportion of caffeinated coffee used. (The following schedule for detoxification, which I use in my practice, is recommended in the book *Caffeine Blues* by research and clinical nutritionist Stephen Cherniske, M.S.)

Days 1-4 Use ¾ regular coffee to ¼ herbal or decaffeinated
Days 5-8 Use ½ regular and ½ herbal or decaffeinated
Days 9-12 Use ¼ regular and ¾ herbal or decaffeinated

Over the next few days, gradually phase out the caffeinated coffee altogether. If you want a "replacement," look in your health food store for herbal coffee or grain coffee substitutes. Postum®, Caffree®, Roma®, Pero®, and Teecino® are some of the more common brands. Some are instant and some are intended to be brewed.

For Tea Drinkers

Although most tea has less caffeine than coffee on a volume for volume basis, it's still caffeine and the same principles apply to reducing your amounts. Brew your tea for less time. Alternate herbal or decaffeinated teas with your cups of black tea. Although green tea is caffeinated, many brands blend green and herb teas, which reduces the amount of caffeine you get in each cup. Gradually reduce your caffeine intake over a two-week period, aiming to be caffeine-free at the end of two weeks.

For Caffeinated Soft Drink Consumers

Your task is to cut down both sugar and caffeine. A good substitute for soft drinks is to mix "fizzy water" (such as Cap-10®) with natural fruit juice. Remember that fruit juice still provides a fair amount of sugar with no fiber, and carbonated beverages of any kind deplete calcium, so this should be viewed as a temporary solution or an occasional treat. Alternate your regular soft drink with one of these fruit juice spritzers. After the first week of this program, begin replacing some of your regular soft drinks with a noncaffeinated soft drink. Ultimately your goal is to eliminate regular soft drink consumption, substituting herbal iced teas or blends of a small amount of fruit juice with herbal tea or water.

INCREASING WATER INTAKE

Often my clients will react to the idea of weaning off soft drinks, coffee, and caffeinated tea with the protest "But what will I drink?" The answer? Water. Water may not be as sexy as drinks that pack a lot of sweetness, buzz, or mouth appeal, but we're talking about health here, not surface image. If health is your priority, water is definitely the beverage of choice.

HOW MUCH WATER DOES *YOUR* BODY NEED?

Figure out the appropriate amount of water for your weight using the ½ ounce per pound of body weight formula. While you may not reach that goal right away, create a plan for working toward that goal. Try to increase your daily amount of water by a glass (8 ounces) per week. Buy one or two water bottles you like and get in the habit of carrying them around. If you drink soft drinks, start replacing some of them with water. Keep track of how much water you drink every day so it becomes more conscious. One strategy I have used is to each morning fill up water bottles equivalent to my daily intake goal. Then it's pretty clear how much I still need to drink without having to think about it.

MOVING FORWARD

THE MAGIC OF SLEEP

As life has gotten busier over the last two decades, Americans are steadily getting less sleep. We have come to see sleep as expendable, as wasted time, even a luxury. Sometimes people report with pride how little sleep they can "get away with." I have fallen into this last category myself, feeling that being "more productive" was somehow a valuable personal quality, never mind that it was at the expense of my overall emotional and physical well-being.

We have a biological need for sleep and rest. It is during this time that our body restores and repairs itself. Our nervous system recoups, our immune system prepares for the next day's work, muscles and tissue repair themselves. Our brain and mind gets a much-needed break from concentration and mental activity that in turn rejuvenates our creativity. Have you ever noticed that taking a break from a mentally demanding task and doing something relaxing or mindless actually increases your effectiveness when you return to the task? Sleep is one way we have of giving our brain the "down time" it needs. Yet most of us sleep on an average only six and a half hours a night.

The use of stimulant-containing food, beverages, and medications often diminishes the quality of sleep people get. Even if it doesn't cause insomnia, caffeine prevents us from going into the deeper stages of sleep known as REM (rapid eye movement). This adverse effect occurs even with caffeine consumed earlier in the day. Alcohol can help you fall asleep, but more than a small quantity in the evening before bed can cause later awakening. Stress often keeps people from falling or staying asleep. The lack of sleep and associated fatigue can keep you in a vicious cycle of using caffeine to stay alert, which then only further promotes fatigue.

When you remove caffeine from your diet, it's also important to pay attention to your changing sleep needs and habits. Sleep is necessary to help the body recover from the damaging effects of chronic caffeine use. And, you will find as you no longer use caffeine to override your fatigue, you simply need more sleep.

Here are some suggestions to help you improve your sleep quality and sleep habits:

1. Establish regular routines. Studies show the same number of hours of sleep is qualitatively better when regular bedtimes are observed over erratic bedtimes.

2. Avoid eating large evening meals or snacking late at night. (Ideally the largest meal should be during the midday.) The digestive fires of the body fade as the day wears on, and nighttime is a time for rejuvenation and repair, not digestion. Heavy evening meals and late snacks interfere with sleep that is refreshing and restorative.

3. Make it a habit to be in bed by 10 PM. If you tune in to your body, you will notice that drowsiness usually sets in between 7 and 9 PM. When you override the natural inclination toward sleep, and stay up later to watch television, or work, the body enters a new phase of increased stimulation. This makes getting to sleep more difficult, and sleep less restful.

4. Stop doing stimulating mental activity at least an hour before bed and begin a wind-down routine. This may include a warm bath, herbal tea, light reading (nothing action-packed or requiring too much concentration), calming audiotapes, or anything else that begins to slow you down. Use dim lighting at this time to help slow down your body and mind.

5. Avoid exercising in the late evening. While regular exercise promotes deep sleep, stimulating aerobic exercise or strength training too close to bedtime will have the opposite effect. Relaxing routines, such as yoga or stretching, are fine.

6. Make sure your room is dark when you go to sleep. Streetlights, moonlight, and even the light from digital clocks keeps your brain from efficiently producing the hormone melatonin, which is produced only in total darkness. Melatonin signals your body to go into deep, healing sleep.

7. If you nap, take either a short one of twenty to thirty minutes or a long one of an hour and a half. If you nap and wake up after thirty minutes and before ninety, you will be interrupting a deeper sleep cycle, which will cause you to feel irritable and more fatigued than not napping at all.

8. There are several natural, nonaddicting sleep aids you can use to help you sleep if you're having difficulty. Since all insomnia does not have the same root cause, I find having several different aids in my natural medicine cabinet is ideal, so I can pick the remedy that is most appropriate for the situation.

NATURAL SLEEP AIDS

Valerian Root Tincture is an herbal preparation that promotes relaxation and will not leave you groggy the next day. Use a dropperful in a glass of water about an hour before bed.

Calmes Forte® is a homeopathic tablet that is especially good when a busy mind is keeping you awake.

GABA is an amino acid that promotes relaxation in both the brain and the gut. Caffeine actually inhibits your body's ability to produce GABA, so if you've been a caffeine user, you are likely short on it. Noncaffeine users may be short on GABA as well. Purchase GABA in a sublingual (under-the-tougue) tablet only because it is destroyed in the stomach by the digestive process and will not be as effective in a cap or caplet form. A sublingual form will send it directly to your brain.

Melatonin is the hormone naturally produced in your brain (see page 133) and can be purchased in tablet form. The 5mg dosage given on bottle labels is usually higher than is necessary and could leave you feeling groggy the next morning. Try a dosage of 1 to 3 mg an hour before bed.

Aromatherapy Oils in a warm bath can be very helpful. Lavender is a particularly relaxing scent, but look for various blends.

Eye Pillows are small beanbags filled usually with flaxseeds scented with lavender. Place them over your eyes for both darkness and the relaxing scent.

IMPROVING YOUR SLEEP QUALITY AND QUANTITY

Pick one or two of the strategies on pages 148 and 149 for improving your sleep and begin to put them into practice. Sweet Dreams!

CHAPTER SIX

HORMONE BALANCE AND IMBALANCE— THE BIG EIGHT

W hen the discussion turns to hormones, people often think only of sex hormones. But your body produces over 150 different kinds of hormones that regulate almost every function of your organism. Hormone imbalance is becoming a larger health issue, in part due to greater awareness of the relationship between the endocrine system and health. But the endocrine system is also affected by diet, toxic exposure, stress, and medication use. In this chapter, we will discuss eight hormones, which if out of balance can produce common symptoms of poor health. Those eight include:

- Insulin
- Thyroid
- Estrogen
- Progesterone
- Testosterone
- DHEA
- Melatonin
- Cortisol

UNDERSTANDING YOUR BODY

I usually suggest that women in their forties and beyond and anyone having chronic health problems discuss hormone testing with their health practitioner. Hormone imbalances are frequently the culprit of, or at least a contributor to, many health problems. Having a baseline reading can provide valuable information as one ages, whether experiencing trouble or not. Within the discussion for each type of hormone below, I've included some testing information so you can go to your health practitioner able to discuss your needs and ready to understand what various tests and test results mean. For most of the hormones discussed, saliva testing is available in home-testing kits. Saliva testing is usually less costly and less invasive than blood testing, it's accurate, and it doesn't require a doctor's prescription. We'll also talk in this chapter about natural and synthetic hormone supplementation.

INSULIN

In Chapter One we discussed the importance of blood sugar regulation in order to control insulin levels. Remember that insulin is the hormone secreted by the pancreas that assists in moving glucose from your bloodstream into your cells. Insulin is released in proportion to your blood-sugar level, so a higher blood-sugar level means greater amounts of insulin. As you know, controlling blood-sugar level through diet is the most effective and noninvasive way to regulate insulin levels and prevent the occurrence of insulin resistance, hyperinsulinemia, hypoglycemia, and diabetes. Keeping insulin levels in the low-to-moderate range also aids in the body's ability to burn both dietary and stored fat and can reverse elevated cholesterol and blood pressure. For reasons that are not yet clear, keeping blood-sugar levels well-regulated seems to help many other health problems, such as gastric reflux, fibromyalgia, chronic fatigue, polycystic ovary disease, and hypothyroidism.

Testing

Although blood insulin levels can be tested, testing blood-glucose levels is an effective and inexpensive way of diagnosing problems with blood sugar regulation. The common *Fasting Blood-Glucose Test* is done by drawing blood after you have fasted overnight for at least eight hours. A normal fasting blood sugar result should be in the 80 to 100mg/dl range. This would indicate that your body had effectively utilized all the carbohydrates you had eaten before the fasting period. If you have not been eating and your blood-sugar level was greater than about 105, I would suspect some level of carbohydrate intolerance.

Although a diagnosis of diabetes usually isn't made until fasting blood-sugar levels exceed 120 to 140mg/dl, significant trouble can be brewing below that level. A person could be insulin-resistant for years before the disease evolves into clinically diagnosed diabetes, years during which many other related health problems could develop and could be halted through lifestyle changes. Elevated blood pressure, elevated triglycerides, low HDL cholesterol, elevated insulin levels, hypoglycemia, and increasing weight with a resistance to weight loss are all likely predictors of insulin resistance and suggest a prediabetic state.

Because of scheduling conflicts, sometimes a blood-glucose test will be done in the afternoon after only a four-hour period of fasting. However, the National Institutes of Health determined these tests to be less accurate. Generally they show a lower blood-glucose level than the overnight fasting test, resulting in a possible missed diagnosis.

A second, more involved test called a **Glucose Tolerance Test** can be done to give a more detailed picture of how well your body is handling carbohydrates. For this test, you are instructed to eat a high-carbohydrate diet for a twenty-four hour period prior to the test. The test involves drinking a high glucose solution after which your blood is drawn at regular intervals for several hours. What your doctor is looking for is a picture of how high your blood sugar gets over time and how long it stays elevated before returning to the normal range of 80 to 100mg/dl.

Both of these tests can also be used to diagnose hypoglycemia, although usually you will know by your symptoms of fatigue, headache, shakiness, indecisiveness, irritability, or lightheadedness, whether you are experiencing hypoglycemia.

There are two types of hypoglycemia: fasting and reactive. Fasting hypoglycemia occurs when, after not eating for a prolonged period (eight or more hours), a person's blood sugar drops too low and he or she feels poorly (not just hungry). Remember learning in Chapter One that your body stores glucose in the form of glycogen for times when you don't have food? That means, after not eating for eight hours, your body, unless you have fasting hypoglycemia, should still be able to maintain a baseline blood-sugar level. With reactive hypoglycemia, your blood sugar drops too low in response to eating a meal that raised it high; this type of hypoglycemia usually occurs within an hour or two after a meal.

THYROID

An underfunctioning thyroid can cause many symptoms, including:

depression	thinning hair or hair loss	brittle nails
obesity	PMS	poor memory
hypoglycemia	inability to lose weight	ovarian cysts
headaches	fatigue	eczema
migraine	fibrocystic breasts	acne
high cholesterol	atherosclerosis	psoriasis
feeling cold often	menstrual difficulties	increased LDL
cold extremities	prolonged morning sluggishness	

An underfunctioning thyroid, especially among women, is commonly unrecognized by doctors. The thyroid hormone affects every system of the body and often symptoms of hypothyroidism are attributed to other causes, or sometimes even discounted. It's not uncommon for a woman to be told her symptoms are related to menopause, or for the doctor to simply write her a prescription for an antidepressant. One out of five women has an underfunctioning thyroid and women are seven times more likely than men to be hypothyroid. Thyroid problems become more likely as one gets older.

Could hypothyroidism be behind your health problems? Certainly if you have any of the symptoms above it is worth considering the possibility. One important thing to do is assess your *risk factors* for thyroid disease. These include a family history of thyroid problems, gender, age, hormonal changes (for women, post-partum and menopausal changes can trigger a change in thyroid function), and personal or family history of autoimmune diseases such as lupus, multiple sclerosis, or rheumatoid arthritis. A very simple way of beginning your personal investigation is to perform the basal metabolic temperature test described below. Then find a sympathetic and knowledgeable doctor to help you proceed.

Testing

Current endocrinology research suggests that the traditional methods of testing and interpreting test results are often ineffective at identifying hypothyroidism and only catch a small proportion of cases.

The standard tests given to determine thyroid function are the TSH or Thyroid Stimulating Hormone test and the T4 test. "T4" stands for Thyroxine, which is the *inactive* form of the thyroid hormone. Thyroxine must be converted to T3 in order to have any effect. If TSH is high, it indicates the thyroid is overworking to produce enough hormone, a sign of an underactive thyroid. However, T4 is the inactive form of the hormone and has to be converted to T3; if there is a problem with the conversion process, a person could be hypothyroid and still have normal-appearing TSH and T4 results.

Many physicians feel the current ranges for the values of TSH tests are too narrow. Some, such as Elizabeth Lee Vliet, author of *Screaming to Be Heard: Hormonal Connections Women Suspect and Doctors Ignore,* believe any person may have a specific TSH at which he or she feels best, and it may not correspond with the averages on the charts.

THYROID SELF-ASSESSMENT

One method of testing you can do yourself is done with a regular, old-fashioned mercury thermometer. This test assesses what your basal metabolic temperature is—the temperature of your body when at complete rest. A low BMT is *highly predicative* of hypothyroid and frequently indicates the condition when it is subclinical and long before standard testing will detect it. Follow the procedure below.

- Use a basal thermometer (the kind with mercury that goes under the tongue). Take your temperature by placing the thermometer under your armpit.

- Do this for five consecutive mornings, as soon as you wake up—don't sit up or move around. Have the thermometer on your nightstand the night before, shaken down and ready to go. Add up the numbers and divide by five for your average temperature.

- Menstruating women should take their temperature beginning with the second day of a period. This point in the cycle gives the most accurate basal metabolic temperature. For men and postmenopausal women, any five consecutive mornings are okay.

- The normal range is 97.8-98.2 degrees Fahrenheit. (Your early morning temperature is slightly lower than your "normal" temperature once you're moving.) If your five-day average is below this, it may indicate a hypothyroid condition and you should check with your doctor. Realize, though, that not all doctors know of this test or of the fact that blood tests may give inaccurate results.

When you have blood work done for thyroid function, request TSH, T4, and T3. Usually a doctor will request the first two, but not T3. If your doctor is not aware of more current information regarding thyroid and thyroid testing, and is not open to learning more, find a doctor who is, as your health may depend on it. An excellent on-line information source for you or your doctor is **www.about.com**. Once on the site, click on the link for health and fitness, then the link for diseases and conditions, then the link for thyroid disease.

ESTROGEN

Estrogen is a family of hormones, not one hormone as is commonly thought. These hormones are primarily produced by the ovaries. We don't yet know the functions of every type of estrogen. The three we know the most about are estradiol, estriol, and estrone. Estradiol is the most predominant. Of these three types of estrogen, estradiol accounts for about 80 percent of the total amount of estrogen produced by a woman's body throughout her life. It is produced from puberty to menopause and is the form of estrogen most related to events such as PMS, peri-menopause, and menopause. Estriol, produced during pregnancy, and estrone produced by fat cells, each account for 10 percent of estrogen

Symptoms of low estrogen familiar to most women (and those close to them!) include moodiness, depression, water retention, hot flashes, and poor memory. The emotional roller coaster connected with estrogen is largely linked to the neurotransmitter serotonin, discussed in "Good Meals, Good Mood." Serotonin levels are tightly linked with estrogen levels, and when estrogen levels decrease, as they do premenstrually and heading into menopause, serotonin levels decrease as well. You'll remember that serotonin helps produce calm, optimistic, clear thinking and the lack of it can make life, well, from a little trying to downright bleak.

Emphasizing foods that boost serotonin can help, as well as following the dietary guidelines emphasized throughout this book. Serotonin-boosting foods are those that contain high amounts of the amino acid tryptophan, such as white meat turkey and chicken, pork, ground beef, Cheddar cheese, tuna, tempeh, cottage cheese, salmon, almonds, lentils, eggs, kidney beans, and milk. Although some books recommend chocolate for boosting serotonin, I don't, because of its effect on blood sugar and glucose and its potential for triggering carbohydrate and sugar cravings.

Estrogen Replacement

As menopause approaches, it's quite common for doctors to give women a prescription for estrogen replacement, rather than engage in an open, informed discussion of all the options. Here are some things you may want to know when considering hormone replacement therapy (HRT):

1. One of the big "selling" points for HRT is that it supposedly reduces a woman's risk of heart disease. The National Women's Health Network is a women's health advocacy group that has reviewed the many studies from which this conclusion was drawn and which were frequently funded by drug companies. The NWHN survey concluded that women who choose hormone replacement therapy tend to be healthier *before* beginning HRT, and therefore are less likely to get heart disease anyway. In fact, women with a higher risk of heart disease or with a history of it are advised *against* the use of estrogen replacement because there is a risk of blood clots and hypertension associated with HRT. All of the lifestyle changes discussed throughout this book will significantly lower your risk of heart disease.

2. Estrogen is frequently prescribed to "prevent osteoporosis." Osteoporosis, or thinning of the bones, raises the risk of bone fracture. In the osteoporosis conversation, we tend to focus on the issue of bone loss. But what rarely is talked about is the *lack of bone formation* that contributes to having weak bones or the dietary factors that contribute to bone loss. Your bones naturally are constantly dissolving and rebuilding. But there are many factors in the standard American diet that contribute to a net bone loss:

   - High sugar intake
   - Use of carbonated beverages
   - Foods that interfere with calcium absorption
   - Inadequate calcium intake from *useable* sources

   We'll go into more detail about these things in the Nutrition Magic section of this chapter. The important point is that calcium loss is within *your* control and is not primarily a function of estrogen deficiency. It is true that estrogen slows down bone loss. So can changing your diet.

And equally important is the other side of the equation—bone forma-tion. Weight-bearing exercise and resistance or strength training are essential for creating bone mass. The loss of bone mass is not so much a function of aging as it is a function of becoming less active either through choice or illness. Becoming more sedentary is, unfortunately, a choice many women either consciously or unconsciously make as they age. We'll address this in Moving Forward.

3. Estrogen replacement is linked with an increased risk of breast cancer. A review of fifty-one studies involving over 52,000 women in twenty-one countries found that women who remained on estrogen replacement for over five years had a 35 percent increase in breast cancer risk.[1]

4. Studies show that women who use estrogen replacement are more likely to develop endometrial and ovarian cancer than women who do not use hormones.

The commonly prescribed hormone replacements are synthetic forms of estradiol and/or estrone. Both of these forms of estrogen are linked with the estrogen-based cancers. Estriol is the one form of estrogen that does not stimulate breast tissue and is anticarcinogenic, yet it is not included in estrogen replacement preparations.

Alternative Treatments

Hormone replacement therapy is not a woman's only alternative for dealing with depression, mood swings, bone loss, hot flashes, or other complications of menopause. Nutrition, supplements, herbs, and exercise can all help promote health and vitality and eliminate problematic symptoms, without the risks and side effects of hormone replacement. Often emotional changes in menopause coincide with other life changes or with unresolved emotions rising to the surface more. This may be a time when more solitude, support, and self-reflection are needed instead of drugs. Hormone

---

[1] Collaborative Group on Hormonal Factors in Breast Cancer, "Breast Cancer and Hormone Replacement Therapy," Lancet 1997; 350; 1047-1059.

replacement is a more invasive level of intervention. Although some women may prefer a pill to eliminate symptoms, for those who want to try more holistic alternatives, HRT can be used as a last resort if nonintrusive and less intrusive measures have been tried without success. Even then, natural hormone replacement is available, with far fewer risks and side effects of the synthetic ones typically prescribed.

Many physicians and health practitioners feel that, in general, women suffer from too much estrogen rather than too little. This is due in large part to the exposure we have to significant amounts of "fake estrogens" (xeno-estrogens) present in all plastic material and in toxic waste. Every time we use plastic bags, plastic containers, plastic water bottles, pop bottles, etc., we are exposed to xeno-estrogens being "out-gassed" from these products. We also consume many phytoestrogens or plant-based estrogens in our diet, especially when soy foods are consumed. Many foods now are ""fortified" with concentrated soy isoflavones. Dr. John Lee, author of *What Your Doctor May Not Be Telling You About Menopause* is a leading educator in the area of "estrogen dominance" and has written several books covering the topic.

Testing

Estrogen levels are typically tested by blood tests but many companies now offer a home testing kit for many hormones, including estrogen, that relies on saliva samples. Testing for estrogen levels is used for clinical verification of menopause. As a woman approaches menopause, her body produces increased amounts of follicle-stimulating hormone (FSH). If you still have periods and you have blood drawn for estrogen, note the day of your cycle, since there is a different range of "normal" values depending on what day you are in your cycle.

PROGESTERONE

Progesterone is mainly produced by the ovaries with small amounts coming from the adrenal glands. Although it is mostly a female hormone, men have and need small amounts, just like woman have and need testosterone. PMS, heavy bleeding during menstruation, headaches, endometriosis, menopausal symptoms, fibrocystic breast disease, and osteoporosis can be symptoms of low progesterone levels. Some doctors have found progesterone helpful in treating men with autoimmune diseases and prostate and cardiovascular problems. Low progesterone levels are often present when low thyroid levels exist. One theory about progesterone-related problems is that they are linked to excessive estrogen levels—called estrogen dominance—from over-exposure to estrogen (discussed above).

Synthetic progesterone is often prescribed for menopausal women along with estrogen replacement. Doctors know that giving estrogen without progesterone (called "unopposed estrogen") is unsafe except when a woman has had a hysterectomy. Synthetic progesterone, like all pharmaceutical hormones, is derived from plant or animal hormones that have been chemically altered (to make them eligible for patenting by a drug company— a natural plant cannot be patented and would produce no profit). The problem with synthetic hormones is that they don't exactly fit the receptor sites that cells throughout the body have for specific hormones. (A receptor site is like a ferry boat dock that will only accept a specific ferry boat. Think of a hormone as the ferry boat that must find its own dock to properly unload its cargo.) Because of this, the synthetic hormones can be less effective than the natural form.

Although estrogen has received a lot of attention for its role in preventing bone loss, progesterone actually stimulates bone formation. Dr. John Lee has reported osteoporosis reversing in woman as late as sixteen years past menopause using natural progesterone cream from wild yam in combination with diet and exercise.

Natural Progesterone Cream

One safe, nonprescription alternative to synthetic progesterone, is the use of natural progesterone cream. Progesterone cream is available over the counter in health stores. Also, a very good brand is sold through a company called Arbonne International, which distributes person-to-person. Both men and women can use progesterone cream.

Testing

As with estrogen testing, progesterone levels can be tested through blood or saliva testing. Like estrogen, the reference range for interpreting results varies depending on the monthly cycle.

TESTOSTERONE

This is an androgen, or male hormone, but don't think women don't have or need it! Quite the opposite is true. It's just that in women a little goes a long way. Symptoms of low testosterone include depression, decreased libido, less sound sleep, less dreaming while asleep, decreased bone density, dry or thin skin, hair thinning, and loss of pubic hair. Studies have also shown a relationship between low testosterone levels and coronary heart disease. Cancer chemotherapy can dramatically reduce testosterone levels in both men and women.

As with other hormones, should supplementing be needed, there is both a natural and synthetic form. Sometimes doctors are reluctant to prescribe testosterone for women, feeling it increases their risk for heart disease by offsetting the risk-lowering effect of naturally-occurring estrogen. However, this contradicts the research showing that low testosterone levels are correlated with arteriosclerosis. Dr. David Brownstein, author of *The Miracle of Natural Hormones* writes: "I have yet to see a severe coronary heart disease patient who did not have a significantly depressed testosterone level." This doesn't prove cause, only that some relationship exists between lowered testosterone levels and heart disease.

Another fear on the part of physicians and many female patients is that the use of testosterone will result in the appearance of male secondary sex characteristics, such as increased growth of facial hair, bulking muscles, or a deepening of the voice. These side effects are a very rare occurrence at the low dosages (under 1.25mg per day) proven effective for most women. This hormone can make it easier for women to build muscle (not bulk up) and generally tone their body (although it should not be given for this purpose when there is already a normal testosterone level).

162

Testing

Testing can be done through blood or saliva. However, since testosterone is only available by prescription, it may be more convenient to go through your health care practitioner for testing. Also, if you are taking the hormone, your blood levels should be monitored periodically to make sure you are neither too high nor too low. *Your doctor must order the test for free testosterone.* If "free" is not specified, the test will be for an inactive form of testosterone, which tells you nothing about how much of the hormone is actually working for you. Don't assume your doctor will know this; many simply write "testosterone" on the lab requisition and you will be given and charged for a useless test.

DHEA

Dihydroepiandrosterone (Say that three times fast!) is a natural steroid produced by the adrenal glands. DHEA levels peak at about age thirty and decline steadily thereafter. At age sixty, they are at about 5 percent of their peak. Sometimes DHEA is referred to as an antiaging hormone because the symptoms of low DHEA are often considered (erroneously) to be the inevitable signs of aging. Low vitality, memory loss, decreasing bone density, muscle mass loss, and a decreased ability to handle stress are often indicators of low DHEA levels. Decreased levels of DHEA are typically present with autoimmune diseases, such as lupus, fibromyalgia, Crohn's disease, ulcerative colitis, and multiple sclerosis.

DHEA is available over the counter, but I recommend testing before buying it to make sure it is needed, and again, after supplementing, to monitor blood levels of the hormone. The average dose is 5 to15mg/day.

Testing

Blood or Saliva

MELATONIN

This hormone is usually thought of for its ability to induce sleep. It is produced by a small gland in the brain, the pineal gland usually peaking between 2 and 4 AM for those who sleep rather than work at night. Melatonin needs total darkness to be released. In addition to inducing sleep, melatonin is a major antioxidant and boosts immunity, so this nighttime renewal process is very important to good health. It also helps your body maintain its circadian rhythm, the natural timing of all our systems that are tied to biological rhythms outside of us, such as the phases of the moon, the seasons, and day and night. Like DHEA, melatonin production decreases significantly with age. People who work night jobs often have sleep difficulty and health problems related to the poor production of melatonin. It is important for late-shift workers, whose biological rhythms have been disturbed, to make sure they create darkness when they sleep during the day so the body can produce melatonin.

Melatonin is manufactured from serotonin, which, as you recall, is made from the amino acid tryptophan. So having enough tryptophan-rich protein sources in your diet will aid melatonin production.

This hormone is useful for sleep disturbances and, after late-night exercise, to promote settling down to sleep. It needs to be taken about an hour before bed. To counter jet-lag after flying, take melatonin one to three hours before bed depending on how many time zones were crossed (an hour for each time zone).

Melatonin is available over the counter without prescription. Generally listed label dosages are high and taken in that amount many people will find they are groggy the next morning. Usually a dosage of 1 to 3mg is effective. If you do find yourself groggy the next morning, try a smaller dose.

Testing

Although you can easily measure melatonin levels yourself through saliva testing (it can also be tested through blood tests), most people who supplement with melatonin do so on as-needed basis without risks or ill effects.

CORTISOL

Cortisol, known as the "stress hormone," is produced by the adrenal glands. The adrenal glands are a frequently unrecognized but important part of your anatomy and heath picture. Walnut-sized and sitting atop each of your kidneys, these glands are involved in the production of many hormones but are most known for their involvement in your body's stress response, as was discussed in Chapter Five. When you face any kind of stress, whether it's work pressure, relationship difficulties, any shocking event or accident, or an injury, your adrenals go to work, producing what is classically known as the "fight or flight" response that puts your system in "overdrive."

- First the hormones adrenaline and cortisol are secreted, which rev up the body to meet the real or perceived threat. These hormones also help sustain energy to different parts of the body that may be involved in meeting the stressful situation. Muscles get activated, ready to "fight" or "flee" and the mind becomes alert and focused.

- Breathing picks up and the heart begins to race or pound.

- Blood pressure rises.

- Endorphins, natural painkillers, are released to numb physical or emotional pain.

- Because the body needs all of its energy for facing the threat, anything extraneous such as hunger, sex drive, or the immune system, is shut down. This reserves all energy for the muscles to face physical danger (even though most of our stress today is not physically threatening).

When stress in our life is a persistent condition, cortisol levels remain constantly elevated. Because high cortisol levels interfere with many normal functions of the body, continually high levels cause fatigue, lowered immunity, depression, and an impaired ability of the body to burn fat, among other difficulties. If you think about it, this makes sense; when you have a crisis in your life, you prioritize things differently, right? Your body does the same thing. But what if the crisis never ends, or keeps going for extended periods of time? Your life would begin to fall apart around you. Ongoing stress has the same effect on your health and your body.

Unfortunately, we have far too many stresses in our lives, and all our technology keeps the pace of life moving faster and faster, multiplying stress exponentially. In addition, poor diets, lack of exercise, caffeine, some medications, and toxins are all sources of additional stress that affect adrenal glands and their stress response. For example, highly elevated blood-sugar levels and insulin resistance can trigger the stress response, because this represents a state of emergency to the body. Ritalin and many medications given for treatment of ADD and ADHD also fire up the adrenal glands.

ADRENAL FATIGUE

Like so many other systems of the body, the adrenal glands can only take so much. In many people they begin to get worn down, producing less cortisol and becoming less able to produce hormones of all kinds. So often, adrenal fatigue is an underlying cause of hormone imbalance. Illnesses such as fibromyalgia and chronic fatigue syndrome frequently have adrenal fatigue or exhaustion at their root. People with these illnesses frequently show hormonal imbalances which can result in a multitude of different symptoms as you have seen throughout this chapter. Can you understand why simply taking a medication for a symptom may mask a problem, thereby jeopardizing your health? A holistic approach to health care is much like peeling an onion; addressing one level of a health problem often leads you to a deeper imbalance.

Stress is more than an inconvenience or unpleasant experience in your daily life. Stress that is frequent or continual is literally squeezing the life out of you. And one of the insidious things about stress is that so many of the things we do on a daily basis—the foods we choose to eat, the lifestyle habits we do or don't maintain—send our adrenals into the battle zone.

Testing

Using saliva testing for cortisol gives a good indication of how much the adrenals are working. Saliva testing is more useful than blood tests because saliva samples can be collected over time more easily than blood can. This gives a more accurate picture. Elevated or depressed cortisol levels can be indicative of high stress or compromised adrenal function.

NUTRITION MAGIC

BONING UP ON CALCIUM

A typical discussion of osteoporosis prevention focuses on consuming enough calcium, but it is a mistake to look at calcium intake without considering two other significant issues:

1) whether calcium is absorbed and assimilated
2) other factors in the diet that actually contribute to calcium loss

INCREASING ABSORPTION

Truckloads of calcium will do you no good if your body is unable to absorb it and convert it to bone. Although it is widely promoted by the dairy council and most nutritionists, dairy is not the best dietary source of calcium. Although it's high in calcium, much of that calcium is not absorbed. Cow's milk has roughly a 1:1 ratio of calcium to the mineral phosphorus. Phosphorus binds with calcium and prevents it from being absorbed. Another mineral, silicon, is essential for calcium absorption and may even transmute to calcium itself. Good sources for silicon are strawberries, apricots, parsnips, celery, cucumbers, carrots, dandelion greens, and oats.

In addition to dairy, there are other foods that inhibit calcium absorption because they contain chemicals that bind with it. Grain products and soy foods both contain a substance called phytic acid, which inhibits calcium and other mineral absorption. Fermenting grains by soaking them for twelve or more hours before cooking, and using fermented soy products, such as tempeh or miso (see glossary), can neutralize the phytic acids and prevent this problem. Oxalic acid, another calcium and mineral inhibitor, is found in asparagus, spinach, Swiss chard, sweet potatoes, and rhubarb. Oxalic acid prevents the absorption of the calcium contained *within* those foods, but not calcium present in other food eaten at the same time. Members of the nightshade family, including tomatoes, potatoes, peppers, eggplant, and tobacco, all contain a naturally occurring chemical called solanine, which inhibits calcium absorption.

BONE BROTH

Paul Pitchford, in *Healing with Whole Foods,* recommends a mineral-rich formula for improving teeth, bones, arteries, and connective tissues and for increasing calcium metabolism. All of these ingredients should be available at a health food store, especially one that sells medicinal herbs.

1 part horsetail (extremely high in silicon)
1 part oatstraw
1 part kelp powder
⅓ part lobelia

Steep 1 ounce of plant material in one pint water for 25 minutes (boil water, turn off heat, add plant material, cover, and let sit). Strain. Drink ½ cup two to three times a day. Use three weeks on, then one week off.

Don't worry about remembering all of these facts right now. You can always come back here and refresh your memory when you are ready to implement some new changes. The most important thing to remember is that there is more to the picture than how much calcium you take in. Total avoidance of calcium-binding foods is not necessary; just be aware of the impact various foods have on your calcium intake, and plan your meals with that knowledge. As usual, eating a wide variety of whole foods is best.

DECREASING DEMINERALIZATION (BONE LOSS)

On the other side of the equation is the issue of bone loss. Bone is live tissue and as such is constantly forming and dissolving. Ninety-nine percent of the body's reservoir of calcium is stored in the bones. If your diet does not supply enough calcium to meet the needs of the heart, muscles, and the nervous system, bone demineralization occurs to supply the deficit. The key issue here is to make sure you aren't losing more bone than is forming. There are many foods that may be a frequent part of your diet that contribute to bone demineralization:

1. Concentrated Sugars: All sugars, including honey, maple syrup, brown rice syrup, turbinado, molasses, etc., cause the blood to become too acidic. When this happens, one way the body neutralizes this acid is by pulling calcium out of bones and teeth.

2. Protein: Protein is often said to increase calcium excretion (measured in urine) and this, in turn, is commonly used as support for a vegetarian diet or to criticize lower carbohydrate diets. Animal protein does, in fact, increase your blood's acidity and will cause demineralization if your diet doesn't neutralize the acidity in some way. What isn't talked about is that the typical meat eater is also eating a lot of grain, breads, sugars, and fats, which also cause the blood to be acidic. Lots of vegetables provide the perfect balancing food for animal protein to prevent calcium excretion. In addition, the green leafy vegetables in particular, such as kale, collard greens, broccoli, and bok choy, all contribute large amounts of absorbable calcium to your diet.

3. Caffeine, Alcohol, Salt: Caffeine, as we discussed in Chapter Five, causes calcium to be excreted in the urine rather than absorbed. When sodium intake exceeds about 1½ teaspoons a day, calcium is lost through urine. The most dramatic loss is shown with alcohol, which interferes with absorption. Social drinkers were shown to have 2½ times the risk of osteoporosis as nondrinkers.

8. Carbonated Beverages: Phosphates (the stuff that gives carbonated beverages their fizz) bind with calcium, inhibiting absorption. This is true even if the beverage is unsweetened, such as the popular "fizzy waters." However, note that sugar-laden carbonated drinks give a double whammy in terms of bone loss.

NONDAIRY SOURCES OF CALCIUM

(suggested daily intake for women is 1200mg)

Green Vegetables (cooked amount = 1 cup)

Lamb's Quarters	516mg	Dandelion Greens	146mg
Bok Choy	330mg	Broccoli	129mg
Collard Greens	304mg	Chard	121mg
Turnip Greens	252mg	Parsley	78mg
Mustard Greens	196mg	Romaine Lettuce	45mg
Kale	178mg		

Other good sources of calcium

Canned Salmon (with small edible bones)	Canned Sardines
Almonds, Hazelnuts, Sesame Seeds	Canned Mackerel
Sea Vegetables—Hiziki, Arame, Wakame	Legumes

PLANNING FOR INCREASED CALCIUM INTAKE

Take stock of the ways your diet may be creating calcium loss. Look over the list of Nondairy Sources of Calcium above. Identify several foods you like and look through the recipes in the back to find some recipes that use those foods. See if you can begin to incorporate high absorption calcium foods in your diet every day.

CONTROVERSIAL SOY

Soy and soy isoflavones have rocketed to the top of everyone's list of "magic bullet" foods in recent years. For vegetarians, tofu and other soy foods often make up a large percentage of protein in the diet. Tofu is encouraged as a heart-healthy meat alternative for nonvegetarians as well. But many studies indicate a darker side to soy that hasn't gotten much press.

Soy contains potent substances, called isoflavones, which mimic estrogen in the body. Because of that, many doctors and nutritionists recommend frequent consumption of tofu, soy milk, soy cheese, and other soy-based products. The claim is that soy will help lower cholesterol, protect against cancer, and help reduce symptoms of both PMS and menopause. Infant soy formula is often used when a nonbreast-fed infant has a dairy allergy.

In the spirit of "if a little is good, a lot is better," isoflavone supplements and enhanced foods are becoming both popular and profitable. But now even leading advocates are urging caution in the use of isoflavone supplements. And many researchers are questioning the consumption of high levels of soy foods especially by postmenopausal women.

What the issue boils down to is the potential harm caused by frequent ingestion of an estrogen-mimicking substance. Although the soy supplements, because of their concentration, pose more of a risk than soy food, regular use of soy foods may put a person at risk as well. A variety of studies have demonstrated a relationship between soy consumption and disruptive effects on thyroid function, a decrease in fertility, and impaired cognitive function. A study of mice, into whom human breast cancer cells were implanted, showed a trend toward larger tumors as the amount of soy in the diet increased.

Japanese researchers have long known that soy has a disruptive effect on thyroid function and believe when given to children, it may pose a risk of thyroid disease later in life.

Long-term data (thirty-plus years) from 7,000 men in a prospective epidemiological study in Hawaii showed an association between consistently high levels of tofu consumption in midlife and low cognitive test scores. Another measurement in the same study found a 2.4-fold increase in Alzheimer's disease in later life in those who ate tofu two or more times a week compared to those reporting little tofu consumption. Three hundred autopsies performed on study subjects from this group showed greater brain shrinkage in those who had consumed higher amounts of tofu. These are fairly alarming pieces of data which deserve more attention and certainly further study.

Because soy foods have become such big business (75 percent of all manufactured food contains soy), the FDA is not likely to look more critically at soy until the weight of evidence and consumer pressure forces the issue.

If soy is a regular part of your or your family's diet, I encourage you to inform yourself about this issue. I recommend the following sources of information:

Soy Online Service **www.soyonlineservice.co.nz**

Weston A. Price Foundation **www.westonaprice.org**

MOVING FORWARD

STRENGTH BUILDS HEALTH

In Chapter Four, "Jumpstarting Your Metabolism," we talked about the role of aerobic exercise in lowering your set point and increasing your metabolism. Now we'll look at the importance to your overall health of building strength.

Strength training, or resistance training as it's sometimes called, is the process of increasing muscle strength through repetitive, weight-bearing movement. Usually the resistance is a weight or a wide elastic band. Sometimes at the beginning of a training regimen, if a person hasn't been exercising or is rehabilitating an injury, no weight is used at all; in this case, body weight provides enough resistance.

Weight training has numerous benefits to overall health above and beyond the vanity aspects so heavily promoted in magazines and on TV.

1. Bone Strength—Weight-bearing and resistance exercise helps promote the formation of bone, increasing bone density and reducing risk of osteoporosis.

2. Fat Burning—Muscle tissue produces enzymes that help with fat-burning. More muscle means greater fat-burning potential, which lowers the set point and helps to burn stored fat.

3. Core Strength—Strength training done properly increases core strength. Core strength refers to the muscles that support the torso—abdominal muscles and those of your middle and lower back. Core strength is essential to support the functional activities of life, such as getting up

out of chairs, sitting up straight, or lifting and carrying heavy objects without incurring injury. Core strength is also necessary for safe and enhanced sports performance.

4. Injury Prevention—Strength training helps prevent slips, falls, and other injuries because strengthened ligaments and tendons do a better job of stabilizing joints. Balance and coordination improve, and the ability to catch oneself before a fall occurs is strengthened.

5. Confidence—Strength training increases confidence and competence. Men and women alike feel better about their bodies and themselves as they gain strength. Many tasks of life become easier when people find they can do things they may not have previously been able to do.

I had one client who, when she first came to see me, had over 100 pounds to lose. After her nutritional program got underway, she began a walking program, then shortly after added very simple strength training at home. Soon, despite her extra weight, she was motivated to go to a neighborhood park basketball court to shoot hoops! Although she had been a basketball player in college twenty years before, knee problems and being out of shape kept her from playing—in fact, kept her from any exercise at all. She had very poor balance and coordination and was always concerned about falling and injuring herself. But within a couple months of walking and strength training, she was able to enjoy a sport that had once given her a lot of pleasure—without fear of injury!

AGING AND STRENGTH TRAINING

Without engaging in regular exercise, including strength training, you will progressively lose muscle mass and lower your metabolic rate in small increments, year by year. The idea that your metabolism slows down as you age, or that the elderly become frail. are really statements about what commonly happens to people, rather than what is a natural part of the aging process. The statements only become true as people stop taking care of themselves and lead a sedentary life.

I mentioned five physical benefits of strength training above. But on a more practical level, let's talk about some of the ways strength training can add to your well-being as you age. Strength training can reduce the pain from arthritis by increasing joint lubrication and nourishment. It can reduce lower back pain and injuries by strengthening related muscles. Reaching, lifting, carrying all become easier with improved flexibility and muscle strength. As sedentary people age, some common problems occur that threaten independent living—climbing stairs, rising from and sitting down in chairs, reaching for things, getting in and out of cars—are a few examples. Loss of hand strength makes opening jars or using tools harder or impossible. All of these gradual losses to health and independance can be avoided and, in many cases, reversed with a very simple program of weight training.

GETTING STARTED

You do not need fancy equipment or even a gym to strength-train. A personal trainer I know shows her clients how to use household objects, such as cans of vegetables, as weights and chairs, walls, and tables as "equipment" for working out. Parents of young babies can even use their infant as a weight, although I don't recommend this practice after feeding your child!

Working out correctly is important to get the most out of your time, to focus on specific needs of your body, and to avoid injury. For this reason, I suggest having at least a few initial sessions with a personal trainer. While it once was considered a luxury to have one, personal trainers now provide valuable instruction to anyone who wants to enhance his or her health. Most trainers will be happy to work with you to help you set up a program and make sure your movements are correct, then consult with you on an as-needed basis after that. Some people prefer an ongoing relationship for the support and motivation it provides.

Strength training works by actually causing muscle fiber to tear. It is in the repairing of the muscle tissue that muscle mass is increased. For this reason, the rest period between workouts is essential and as important as the workout itself. Often I see new exercisers at the gym doing strength training every day on the premise that if a little is good, a lot is better. But this is definitely not the case with strength training. You should give any muscle group that you worked at least forty-eight hours of recovery time before you work it again.

Some people prefer to rotate working out the upper body muscles with working out the lower body muscles. Others like to do a full body workout at once. The choice is yours, depending on your time, stamina, and other activities. Don't forget strength training should be incorporated into an exercise program that includes aerobic activity. It is fine to do strength training and aerobics on the same day if you have the time and energy to do that. You can vary the order of the two, based on personal preference. You may find you have more energy for the second activity by using a particular order.

Because weight training is a sugar-burning (anaerobic) activity, it uses stored glycogen as its fuel. Remember that depleting glycogen stores is a good thing, because it allows more glucose from the carbohydrates you eat to be stored in the muscle instead of as fat. If you are inclined to do both an aerobic activity and strength training in the same workout, there is one possible advantage to doing the strength workout first. Before your body can go into fat-burning mode during aerobic exercise, it needs to use up circulating glucose first; this is why you always hear that you don't start to burn fat until after twenty minutes of activity (you burn calories but not fat). If you deplete your glucose and glycogen through your strength workout, more of your aerobic workout will actually burn stored fat.

 CHOOSING STRENGTH TO SUPPORT LIFE

Make a list for yourself of what goals you might have for a strength-training program. Are there areas of physical function that you would like to improve? Do you suffer lower back or arthritic pain, or do you have an old injury that bothers you? Do you want to tone your body, improve your flexibility, or increase your metabolism? Are you concerned about osteoporosis?

CHAPTER SEVEN

PRACTICALLY SPEAKING

Okay, you want to be healthier and you're convinced that nutrition is an important piece of your health picture. But:

- You're busy, hate to cook, travel a lot, eat out often, and have a _____ (spouse, kid, fill in the blank) who balks at eating anything slightly resembling a vegetable.

- The people in your office have doughnuts and dishes of candy everywhere, exercise is boring, and besides you leave for work too early and get home too late to fit it in.

- Your mother-in-law, with whom you eat dinner every Sunday, insists on serving carbohydrates à la mode and your husband wonders why you can't cook like his mother.

- Life wouldn't be worth living if you could never eat _____ (fill in the blank) again.

- You feel too tired to do all the things outlined in this book.

Have I left anything out?

I sympathize. Really I do. Every one of us faces some, even most of these situations. The key to your success is whether you look at these difficulties as challenges to be solved creatively or whether you hold them out as excuses. It's all a matter of attitude and your attitude is up to you and only you. In almost every class I teach, there is at least one person who is sarcastic and has witty comebacks to everything I suggest. These people are generally resentful that they *have* to change their diet and how they think about food. If you are reading this book, I will presume that you are an adult. You don't *have* to change your diet; you just need to be willing to live (or die) with the impact your diet has on your health. And, if you are responsible for feeding children, you have some responsibility for their health and for shaping their attitudes toward feeding themselves. If you have decided that you want to be healthier (if you've read this far, I'm guessing you have) and are willing to change your nutritional style to reach that end, this chapter will offer practical advice for meeting some of the challenges that will come your way as you journey to better health.

ANTICIPATE, ANTICIPATE, ANTICIPATE!

Did I mention anticipation? There are very few eating situations that can not be handled by having healthy food available, if you make the effort to think and plan ahead. Sometimes this requires more effort than other times. Generally, you will find that the more you practice planning, the more second-nature it becomes.

QUESTIONS FOR DAILY PLANNING
- What is your day going to be like in terms of pace, energy demands, time for meals, etc.?
- How often will you need to eat ?
- Where are you likely to be throughout the day, especially at mealtimes?
- What food will be available to you when you do need to eat?
- What steps can you take to make sure healthy food choices are available to you?

THE TRAVELER

People who routinely travel in their line of work have some special challenges when it comes to regulating diet. Typically, the traveler is eating most of his or her meals in restaurants or at luncheons where the food choices may be limited. Also controlling one's meal schedule may be more difficult. Here are some suggestions that have worked for many of my traveling clients to help them gain more control over their food choices while away from home.

1. If your plans involve a hotel stay, phone ahead and request a room re-frigerator. Plan to bring a small, soft-sided cooler with you. You can find these easily in most department stores along with slim "blue ice" packets to keep your food cool. One that is large enough to hold a six pack should give you ample room. No, you are not going to bring a six pack! What you most likely will need to supplement will be your breakfast (in the event your hotel only supplies a continental breakfast of toast, pastry, and juice) and some snacks. Possible items to bring include: small apples, tangerines or oranges, individually wrapped string cheese, deli meat in small plastic bags, baby carrots, cut-up celery, homemade trail mix (see recipe on p.193), nitrate-free beef or turkey jerky.

   If you have a larger breakfast menu available, look for eggs or an omelet and add other healthy carbohydrates as your particular nutritional plan suggests. Plan to keep your tote accessible during the day so you can grab a snack when needed.

2. Conferences and company luncheons can be a bit more difficult since you have very little control over your food choices. Depending on your comfort level you could inquire ahead as to the menu, let the organizer know that you have some medical restrictions, and see if you can make sure there will be something you can eat. A salad alone won't do unless you will have an opportunity shortly before or after to get some kind of protein. As more people express their preferences for healthy carbohydrate choices and adequate protein, the corporate culture will be inclined to change meal choices. All companies are concerned about

their rising health care costs and you are actually performing a service by encouraging them to make the connection between their meal planning, employee health, and their bottom line.

If you are unable to secure an adequate meal for yourself at a business function, use your personal "stash" of food to provide you with adequate protein before, during, or after the function as is comfortable for you. Remember that your health is a cause worthy of making a few ripples.

3. If you are a sales rep or consultant who drives a lot in your job, purchase an inexpensive soft-sided lunch container for your car. Keep it in your car and stocked with nonperishable protein sources, such as nitrate-free beef or turkey jerky, protein snack bars, small "pop-top" cans of tuna (these have very little juice and can easily be eaten without a mess), and some nuts. You might include a package of low-glycemic 100 percent rye crackers, such as Finn Crisp®, Wasa®, or Rye-Vita®. Also throw in a plastic fork and a few napkins or moist towelettes. You can supplement this packet with portable fruits and vegetables on individual trips. This car pack will help you avoid getting stuck being hungry or having low blood sugar with no option other than minimarts or fast food joints. They can also save you on a long commute home that stretches you beyond "slightly hungry" and into "ravenous."

RESTAURANT EATING

Dining in restaurants doesn't usually pose the problem most people imagine. Generally, it is possible to find meat, fish, eggs, or poultry on the menu along with salads and vegetables. (If you are a vegan and eat no animal products, you will probably have a more difficult time finding adequate protein sources that don't also give you an overload of carbohydrates). Unless you are eating with others or you are a masochist, you might ask the waitperson not to leave bread or rolls on your table. Try ordering a salad right away if you are hungry, even before you place your meal order. For dressing in restaurants, it's usually safest to stick with oil-and-vinegar based dressing. Don't be shy about asking if a dressing has added sugar, and if so, pass on it. Blue cheese or ranch are two choices that will be low in carbohydrate but could easily give you an excessive amount of calories from fat if you don't use them moderately. Ask for it on the side and dip your fork in the dressing then into your bite of salad. Also, in most restaurants, be aware that the commercial dressings they serve will most certainly use hydrogenated fats. For all these reasons, an olive oil dressing is your most reliable option.

For your meal, find a protein-based entrée that appeals to you. Things to watch for that may trip you up are:

- sauces that contain sugar or honey (often fruit or teriyaki types)
- breaded or fried anything
- items wrapped in bread, phyllo, pastry, etc. (if you can leave off the wrapping, no problem)
- heavy cream sauces (could be served on side so you can control the portion)

Most restaurants serve potatoes, rice, or pasta as a side dish with entrées, but I have found they are always willing to substitute extra vegetables in place of the refined carbohydrate. In fact, many restaurants are becoming increasingly aware of and responsive to the needs of people trying to limit their refined carbohydrate intake.

Fast food restaurants don't have as many options for healthy eating as sit-down restaurants, but most these days have caught on to some degree. You can almost always find a salad (albeit most of the time an anemic one), and that can be supplemented with protein from their sandwich offerings. Choose a broiled or grilled option over something fried and, of course, skip the bread. Chili in fast food places is usually very high on the carbohydrates and may be a good choice only for those following a "fit and healthy" type plan.

WHEN OTHER PEOPLE PLAN THE MENU

Dinner invitations, potlucks, and parties require as much psychic preparation as food-related preparation. Since most of the world subsists on refined carbohydrates, you usually will be faced with a selection of foods that won't meet your needs. And, in the case of potlucks and parties, unless you mentally prepare ahead of time to do otherwise, you could find yourself easily overeating.

I have a personal rule of thumb when someone invites me to dinner. If it's someone I know well, or someone who inquires as to my food preferences, I let them know that I feel better if I eat primarily protein and vegetables. This generally doesn't present a problem for people. If I do not know the host or hostess well, and they don't ask, I don't obsess about it and I do the best I can. In either case, I usually ask if I can bring a contribution to the meal. If the answer is yes, this gives me an opportunity to ask what the menu will be so I can bring something that fits in and meets my needs as well.

For potlucks and office gatherings, the typical fare will be pasta or rice salads, chips, dips, bread-based items, and sugar. Usually at least one person will bring some cut-up veggies. I have found that most people are incredibly appreciative of a dish that offers more protein or an interesting vegetable combination. Even something as simple as tuna or chicken salad will be a hit. If you bring something like this as your contribution, just make sure you get some because it will likely go fast!

NUTRITION MAGIC

By far the biggest area of change for most people will be in the kitchen, working with the day-to-day food prep. Unless you have the kind of disposable income that will allow you to pay someone else to prepare food for you, be it a store or an individual, there is no escaping the fact that eating healthy will require you to spend some time preparing food at home. This preparation can be kept fairly simple if you don't have time or really don't like to cook. The more time you put into it, the more interesting and varied your meals can be. But you can start simply.

KEEPING A WELL-STOCKED KITCHEN

The one common characteristic shared by people who cook a lot is that they keep a well-stocked kitchen. Having to go out and buy three spices or a can of tomatoes or any list of ingredients each time you want to throw something together is sure to make cooking a time-consuming if not unpleasant experience. Keeping your kitchen well-stocked with the nonperishable ingredients that fit into your nutritional lifestyle can actually make it fun to find and try a new recipe. You may need to stop and pick up the protein needed or a few vegetables, but if you shop regularly for these items and keep some extra meat in your freezer, it's quite easy to limit your shopping to a weekly trip. See the master-shopping list on page 187 to get you started.

You may want to add items to your pantry gradually as you try new recipes. But these are the basic ingredients that will allow you to make almost any recipe in this book. Having a well-stocked kitchen will also allow you to pull a meal out of the hat in a pinch—well, almost!

KITCHEN CUPBOARD MAKEOVER

If you are serious about changing your nutritional lifestyle, let your actions reflect your intention. Devote a block of time to going through cupboards, cleaning out the old and making room for the new. When you clear a block of time for going through your kitchen like this, you are creating psychic as well as physical space. No, this does not mean that you are going to channel disembodied spirits while hanging out in your pantry! There are two levels of change here. One is the change in habits or behavior— doing things like shopping differently, bringing lunch to work instead of buying fast food, or learning to make a sweet dessert without refined sugars. The other is the more organic change in how you will think about and experience food and your body. These changes have more to do with what goes on inside you than with what you do with food.

These two types of change clearly feed each other, but people who are most successful at making permanent, deeply rooted changes focus intentionally on both parts of the process. The internal changes actually promote chemical and physical changes in your organism that support new ways of behaving and thinking. One reason that clearing a block of time for reorganizing your kitchen is so helpful is that it allows your whole being to "get with the program." It's a way, in effect, of saying to all the cells in your body, "Okay, everybody, we're starting a new project and I want everyone's attention and cooperation." It allows you time to consciously or unconsciously process thoughts and feelings connected to your health, your body, your relationship with food, your concerns about making these changes, etc. Whether you're aware of every part of this process is not critical. What's important is only that your whole organism has time to go through it.

THE CLEAN-OUT PLAN

You will need to decide how "pure" you want to be in terms of getting rid of man-made or chemical-filled products. Below are some criteria you may want to apply as you look through your cupboards. If you live with other people who don't share your ideas about nutritional change, you may find it helpful to designate some cupboard space that is yours alone.

#1 Does this food contain damaged or hydrogenated fat?

Likely suspects are crackers, biscuits and biscuit mixes, cookies, mixes for cookies and muffins, most snack foods like chips, pretzels, corn chips, flavored popcorn, commercial brands of granola, pastries, frozen desserts (other than ice cream), and most packaged items that are not fresh food.

#2 Is this food highly processed or does it contain chemical preservatives?

Food in this category would include processed lunchmeat, bacon, and sausage that contains nitrites, nitrates, artificial coloring, BHT, or other carcinogenic chemicals. Highly refined foods include cold cereals, white bread, most baked goods, bagels, pizza crust, pie crust, cornbread, bread sticks, pita bread, pasta, cous-cous, rice noodles, white rice, phyllo dough, tortillas, ice cream cones, rice cakes, pretzels, corn chips, and most crackers.

Also, sugar and most sweeteners or foods that contain them, such as brown sugar, honey, molasses, maple syrup, brown rice syrup, barley malt, pudding and pudding mixes, jams, jellies, chutneys, cakes, pies, candy, cookies, sweet rolls, banana bread, sweetened cocoa mix, ice cream, marshmallows, most peanut butter, most commercial salad dressings, and most low-fat products fall into this category.

#3 Does this food make use of chemical sweeteners?

For many people, use of products with artificial sweeteners causes severe health problems (despite official claims to the contrary). These chemicals also trigger sugar and carbohydrate cravings in many people. Soda pop, ice tea and other cold drink mixes, gelatin desserts, pudding mix, cocoa mix, ice cream and frozen yogurt, frozen desserts, chewing gum, sugar-free syrups, and baked goods are common items that use artificial sweeteners.

#4 Does this food contain MSG?

Monosodium Glutamate (MSG) is very frequently added as flavoring to lots of processed food. It rarely is listed as such on the label, however, making it difficult to detect. Many people are not aware they are sensitive to MSG. Common symptoms of MSG sensitivity include headaches, migraines, stomach upset, nausea and vomiting, diarrhea, irritable bowel syndrome, asthma attacks, shortness of breath, anxiety or panic attacks, heart palpitations, partial paralysis, heart attack-like symptoms, balance difficulties, mental confusion, mood swings, neurological disorders (Parkinson's, MS, ALS, Alzheimer's), behavioral disorders (especially in children and teens), allergy-type symptoms, skin rashes, runny nose, bags under the eyes, flushing, mouth lesions, and depression.

Hydrolysis, a process often used with soy protein, creates monosodium glutamate. If you look at ingredient labels on manufactured foods, hydrolyzed soy protein or hydrolyzed protein is often a major ingredient. You will frequently see this on the thousands of fairly new soy-based vegetarian meat analogs, burgers, textured soy proteins, and protein powders. Even if you don't believe you are sensitive to MSG, some researchers and doctors state that MSG triggers insulin release and is likely part and parcel of the hyperinsulinemia and carbohydrate craving cycle. Certainly, if you suffer from any of the symptoms mentioned above, consider MSG as a possible cause or contributor to the problem. A four- to six-week trial of eliminating MSG from your diet and observing your symptoms could be a worthwhile experiment if you have health problems that have been unresponsive to any other intervention. Although most of the offending foods will probably be on your "to go" list anyway, you may need to avoid some additional items.

Definite sources of MSG include hydrolyzed protein, sodium caseinate or calcium caseinate, autolyzed yeast or yeast extract, and gelatin. Possible sources include textured protein, carrageenan or vegetable gum, many seasoning blends, flavorings or natural flavorings, chicken, beef, pork, or smoke flavorings, bouillon, broth, or stock, barley malt, malt extract, malt flavoring, whey protein, whey protein isolate or concentrate, soy protein, soy protein isolate or concentrate, soy sauce or extract.

This is a huge list and you may choose to eliminate some but not all of these items. As you can tell from the "possible sources" list, MSG is often a hidden ingredient contained in another ingredient; the FDA does not require MSG to be identified as such on a label. If you have chronic health problems for which you cannot identify a source, you will be safest to avoid manufactured food and eat only fresh food.

If you're making nutritional changes on your own in a household of confirmed carbohydrate, sugar, and processed food eaters you will have the challenge of maintaining your focus on your goals and priorities. Many initially disinterested or oppositional spouses become more interested when they notice the rapid and dramatic changes in their partner's energy, mood, appearance, and overall health. So don't assume a resistant partner will stay that way. Among my clients, I have found that kids, especially younger ones, are quite willing to try new food.

Once you have decided which food stays and which food goes, it's time to fill your cupboards, refrigerator, and freezer with fresh, life-giving food. Use the shopping list that follows as a guide for food that is the basis of good taste and good health.

TAKE TWO APPLES MASTER SHOPPING LIST

Pantry

Nut Butters—Peanut, Almond, Sesame
    Tahini, Cashew
Olive Oil, Sesame Oil
Coconut Milk
Vinegars—Brown Rice, Organic Cider,
    Balsamic
Tamari Soy Sauce, wheat-free
Stevia—liquid
Just Whites ® Powdered Egg Whites
Gelatin—unflavored
Extracts—assorted flavors (e.g., Vanilla,
    Maple, Coffee)
Vanilla/Chocolate Whey Protein Powder
Tuna Fish—water-packed Albacore
    (no soy filler)
Canned Salmon
Sardines, Anchovies
Canned or Jarred Beans—garbanzo,
    kidney
Stocks—chicken, vegetable, mushroom
Whole Tomatoes, diced, and Tomato Paste
Rice—wild, short grain, brown
Quinoa
Dried Lentils—green, red, yellow
Sesame Seeds
Rye Vita Crackers®
Wasa Rye Crackers®
Finn Crisp Crackers®
Sprouted Grain Bread (flourless)

Refrigerator

Oils—Peanut, Walnut
Low-fat Plain Yogurt
Low-fat Sour Cream
Mustard—dijon, stoneground, yellow
Horseradish
Mayonnaise—no sugar, good oil
Miso—light and dark
Umeboshi Plum Paste
Salsa
Olives

Raisins
Dill Pickle Relish (no sugar)
Feta and/or Blue Cheese
Parmesan Cheese
String Cheese
Fresh Fruit
Fresh Vegetables (concentrate on low-glycemic fruits and vegetables with some higher-glycemic root vegetables)

Freezer

Frozen Vegetables (avoid pea, corn mixtures)
Frozen Berries
Frozen Bananas
Coconut, shredded, unsweetened
Nuts—Almonds, Walnuts, Pecans, Cashews
Shrimp
Turkey Burgers
Ostrich Sausage and Patties
Boneless Chicken Breast
Cut-up Fryer Chicken
Ground Turkey, Chicken (white and dark)
Lean Ground Beef
Lean Beef (loin or round cuts)
Turkey Breast
Lean Pork (loin cuts)
Fish Fillets and Steaks
Tempeh

For Vegetarians:

Vegetarian Burgers*—18 grams carbohydrate
    or less such as:
Boca Burgers®
Okara Patties®
Morningstar Farms®—some varieties
Lightburgers®
Gardenburgers®

    *Most vegetarian burgers contain MSG in the form of hydrolyzed protein, as well as concentrated soy protein. I don't recommend regular use of these products unless you are a vegetarian and unwilling to eat animal products.

MOVING FORWARD

PROGRESS NOT PERFECTION

Progress not perfection is a saying often used in twelve-step recovery programs. I like it because it speaks to the ongoing nature of change. Most people whom I counsel have been eating less than optimally for some time, maybe even a lifetime. Some are more aware of it than others. The fact is, any change for the better is going to make a difference. It doesn't have to be done all at once. And the best part is, the worse one's diet is now, the more immediate benefit he or she will see from the initial small changes.

If you are feeling all these changes are too big or unmanageable, know that you can change that experience right now simply by reminding yourself as often as necessary that you don't have to do it all at once. Decide on which things you will and can work on changing right now and focus on those. When you feel ready to take another step, take one. You are not doing this for your doctor or your nutritionist or your spouse, you're doing it for you. You must be the one to balance the consequences of whatever dietary decisions you make with the discomfort of changing your eating habits. So make it work for you.

DON'T STOP NOW!

If you're feeling put upon or overwhelmed, take a look at how you are "holding" the idea of this change in your mind. Do you feel as though someone is "making" you do it? If so, where does that belief or feeling come from? What are your reasons for wanting to make changes in your diet?

STAYING FOCUSED ON CHANGE

Review the tasks marked with an apple or a walking puzzle piece in previous chapters. Pick out ones that spoke to you or that you feel are doable. Make a list for yourself and prioritize them, keeping in mind that some of the steps in the first three chapters will give you the most bang for your buck right away, such as eating more protein or starting a walking program.

CHAPTER EIGHT

MAKE IT
HEALTHY, MAKE
IT FAST

I don't love doing laundry or cleaning my house. I hate balancing my checkbook. But doing all of those things with some degree of proficiency is a necessity to take care of myself. I used to just dump all my clothes in the washer at once until a girlfriend taught me about sorting clothes, different water temperatures, and the finer points of soaking and stain removal. I survived just fine with the dump and wash method, but my whites never stayed white and practically every top I owned had some kind of stain on it from food or a pet.

Cooking is also one of those things that I put into the category of an acquired life skill. We aren't born knowing how to cook, even though many people of both sexes still assume there's a female chromosome for it. I was fortunate enough to learn a lot about cooking from my mother, even more fortunate that I love to cook. I suspect my love for it came in part because I learned without pressure, just by hanging out with my mom, a very creative cook, in the kitchen. The other part is simple—I love to eat great food! Those things aside, cooking isn't something that is intuitive for most people, or that comes without some kind of instruction or without practice. And with fewer people cooking today, generations of young people are growing up without a clue of what to do in the kitchen besides tear open boxes and use a microwave.

When I teach cooking classes, I hear from my students how much learning kitchen techniques and tricks transforms cooking from a dreaded task to something that can be enjoyed, if only for the pleasure of eating the results. You may never love to cook, but feeding yourself well is an important life skill. If you don't already know the basics, taking time to learn them can really change your feeling about cooking. Look in local newspapers for cooking classes. Health food stores often sponsor or know of cooking classes, and community or adult education programs often run them as well.

If you have children, get them involved in food preparation. If you don't know how to cook well, take a class with them; most kids love to cook. Younger children find it magical to transform a pile of ingredients into something deliciously edible. You will be giving them skills they need and for which someday they will be grateful. And besides, it will lighten your workload, give you a shared activity, and encourage healthier eating habits. Kids who participate in food preparation are less picky eaters, because they feel some ownership and pride in the food they helped to prepare. They are more likely to try new foods if they have a hand in the decision making about what to cook and how to cook it. Take them shopping, let them plan some meals, use it as an opportunity to discuss food and health with them. Ultimately, changing the health of the nation depends on younger generations understanding where *real* food comes from, and that's not out of a box.

MAKING THE MOST OF YOUR TIME

Lack of time is probably the strongest force against maintaining healthy eating habits. Most people like the taste of healthy food and like the way they feel after eating it. But time pressures can push even the most dedicated person back into the trap of less healthy or downright unhealthy convenience food. The trick to staying on track is making healthy food convenient, and this section is devoted to sharing with you my shortcuts and ideas for doing that.

SHOP REGULARLY

Scheduling time for weekly shopping, if you aren't in the habit of doing that, will help you save time and support healthy eating. Most grocery stores are stocking more fresh foods, packaged for convenience: baby carrots, shredded cabbage, sliced mushrooms, prewashed lettuce, Middle Eastern specialties like hummus and baba ghanouj, roasted chickens, and, of course, sliced deli meats. Yes, you will you pay more for the convenience of prepared food, but you probably will save money by having food available to pack for lunches and snacks instead of buying out, and you'll waste less food that goes bad before you ever cook it. And then there's the obvious benefit to your health!

Keeping your cupboards, refrigerator, and freezer well-stocked (use the master list on page 187) will also make cooking and food preparation in general a lot less of a hassle. I have found that many people who hate to cook really hate the bother that comes from not being well-organized. If you can develop some simple habits and build on them over time, you may find that it's not as bad as you thought. One of my clients told me at our first consultation that she hated cooking, was too busy, and really did not want to have to cook in order to be healthy! We started by having her make simple changes that required minimal kitchen time, but added more protein and vegetables to her diet and deemphasized refined carbohydrate foods. She made protein smoothies in the morning, utilized some of the "quick combo" ideas you'll find in this section for snacks, and broiled a piece of salmon a couple times a week.

Within a week she called, very excited to let me know she had *a* lot more energy, had dropped some weight, and simply felt better all around. It was this dramatic response to eating differently that inspired her to try making a few simple recipes. Then she discovered that she really *liked* having some new and delicious food around and found that after she'd made a recipe once, it didn't take much time to do it the next time. She is still a very busy person, still is not interested in cooking up a storm, but she has found that a small investment of her time to prepare some meals is really paying huge dividends in how the rest of her life goes. She has experienced a tremendous improvement in her health that even her doctor can't believe and has lost over fifty pounds. Even her husband, who previously wanted nothing to do with her healthy food, has now decided he'd like to give her approach a try.

START WITH QUICK COMBOS

Below are some easy, no-cook answers to the question "What should I eat?" Each of these suggestions supplies a meal or snack with a combination of protein, fat, and carbohydrate. Not every suggestion may be appropriate for you. Using the meal plan from Chapter Three that you decided is best for you, you can choose to include, limit, or avoid any food suggestion below, or throughout the rest of this book. For example, someone following the Healing Plan would do best to limit chili, because of the concentration of high carbohydrate beans, or fruits that have a high sugar content. When using pre-made items, check ingredient labels to avoid hydrogenated fats and chemicals.

- cottage cheese, 1 block of fruit, 1 tablespoon chopped nuts or flaxseed meal
- protein smoothie made with 1 block fruit and flaxseed oil or nut butter
- sprouted grain toast with 1 tablespoon peanut or almond butter
- 1 to 2 hard boiled eggs with 1 block fruit or with cut-up vegetables
- tuna salad and apple
- canned lentil soup, store-roasted chicken, cherry tomatoes, baby carrots
- eggless tofu salad, mixed greens salad with dressing
- ham or turkey rolled around string cheese stick, cut-up sweet peppers, cherry tomatoes, apple, orange or kiwi fruit
- canned chili with extra cooked ground beef or turkey, mixed greens, and veggie salad with dressing
- 2 string cheese sticks and pear
- roasted chicken, salad greens (prewashed) with cherry tomatoes, baby carrots, cucumber, 1 tablespoon olive oil and vinegar type dressing
- plain low-fat yogurt with protein powder mixed in, 2 teaspoons fruit-only jam, chopped, toasted nuts

NUT SNACK MIX
1 ½ cups Raw or Tamari Roasted Almonds*
1 cup Raw Cashew Pieces
½ cup Raisins
1 cup Flaked Unsweetened Coconut
serving = ¼ cup (limit to 1 or 2 servings per day)

*Tamari is a wheat-free soy sauce that adds a nice flavor. These almonds are usually available in health food stores that sell bulk items. Avoid any roasted nuts that are roasted in oil because of the added fat.

Other Suggestions:
- Salad bars often have good selections if you avoid the pasta and potato salads and sweetened salad dressings. Make sure to include a good source of protein, such as tuna or chicken salad, diced ham, feta cheese, or hard-boiled eggs. Chickpeas provide both protein and carbohydrate.
- Many larger health food groceries have deli cases with good selections. Look for roasted chicken, turkey meatloaf, sautéed mixed greens, marinated mushrooms, roasted root veggies, and other prepared vegetable dishes. Be aware of foods that use sweeteners or that are primarily pasta or grains. The more of a healing diet you need, the less tolerance you have for these, even in small amounts.
- In restaurants, Greek salads, grilled chicken Caesar salads (leave out the croutons), chicken or fish dishes with sides of steamed veggies are good choices.

COMPONENT COOKING

Component cooking is simply the art of leveraging your time in the kitchen by making or preparing food that can be used in two or more different ways throughout the week. Most people are too busy to fool around with making food that's gone in a single mealtime. Why not use your time to stock your refrigerator with elements that can be turned into several different meals or snacks?

Component cooking requires that you:

1) set aside a block of time to plan what you want to have
2) shop for the fresh ingredients (because you, of course, have stocked your kitchen with all the nonperishables!)
3) cook

It may take you three to four hours a week, but it doesn't have to be all at once. Once you've done it a few times, you'll get faster, you'll get more ideas flowing, and you won't need as much planning time. I will give you some suggestions to get you started, but don't forget that most of the recipes in the back of the book are designed with component cooking in mind. Chapter Nine will also give you some ideas for multiple ways to use the same food.

The other guideline I offer for busy people, especially those who don't care for cooking, is to always cook enough quantity for more than one meal! If it's something that will freeze, so much the better.

Here are some of the basic components:

In-House Salad Bar

Don't you just love a salad bar where you can quickly build a fresh, crunchy salad from piles of ingredients already washed and chopped for you? Why not create one in your refrigerator at home? Many salad items keep well once washed and chopped; others, like lettuce, do better washed, but with leaves kept whole until you're ready to use them (unless you opt for the cellophane bags of prewashed).

Wash, seed, and chop sweet red, orange, yellow, and green peppers. Store in glass jars to keep them fresh four to five days. Wash and chop an entire bunch of green onions to use in salads or as garnishes; they also keep best in a glass jar. Radishes, baby carrots, snow peas, shredded red cabbage, spinach, jicama, daikon radish, grape or cherry tomatoes, sliced mushrooms, and celery are all vegetables that will hold up if you cut them in advance. Lettuce leaves can be washed, dried carefully (a lettuce spinner is great for this), then wrapped in paper towels and stored in a plastic bag or one of the reusable vegetable bags available in produce sections in many stores. Cucumbers tend to dry out if cut in advance, so cut those as needed. (I use the small salad cucumbers because they are not waxed. Be sure to peel waxed cucumbers.)

Salad Dressings can easily be made in advance and most will keep far longer than it will take you to use them up if you eat salad regularly. Make one or two varieties so you don't get bored. I use the Essential Herb Vinaigrette recipe regularly for salads, to marinate steamed vegetables, and as a marinade for chicken or beef.

Steamed or Parboiled Vegetables

Cutting up and slightly cooking vegetables until crisp-tender is the best way I know to get yourself in the habit of eating more vegetables. Are you tired of finding brown mushy plastic bags on the bottom of your vegetable drawer from something you completely forgot about after you brought it home from the store? Steaming or parboiling is the solution.

The idea here is to wash and cut up a variety of vegetables you like or want to try. Be brave and try something you don't usually eat! Once they're cut up, you either lightly steam them one type at a time until crisp tender, or you drop them, again one type at a time, in a couple inches of boiling, salted water (also called parboiling). Leave the pot uncovered with either method so the vegetables don't overcook. Vegetables should be brightly colored and slightly resistant to a prick with a fork or knife tip. Parboiling takes just a minute or two of cooking, steaming a bit longer. Once cooked, remove the vegetables with a slotted spoon or strainer and plunge them in a bowl of ice water in your sink. Chefs refer to this as "shocking" your vegetables! This will instantly stop the cooking and keep the vegetables from becoming mushy. If you're in a hurry, running under cold water will do. Do not throw out the cooking water—reuse it with each new vegetable. When you're done, save the water for soup stock or just as a mineral-rich, warm, vegetable bouillon to drink. You can easily freeze the broth for later use in soup.

Individually steam or parboil any combination of the following vegetables:

Asparagus—Snap off tough lower portions, steam or parboil until bright green

Broccoli florets—Steam or parboil until crisp, barely tender, still bright green

Cabbage—Cut into thin wedges; steam for 4 to 6 minutes

Carrots—Slice with the knife angled diagonally to get this ➡ then steam or parboil

Cauliflower florets—Steam or parboil until crisp, barely tender

Daikon radish— (looks like a huge, white carrot) Slice on the diagonal as for carrots; cook lightly

Green beans—Trim off vine end only; lightly steam until bright green and still crisp

Winter squash—Delicata and dumpling are two varieties of small, very sweet squashes that can be cut into half-circle slices or small wedges and steamed until soft but not mushy. Delicatas can be cut in half horizontally, seeds scooped out, then placed cavity down and sliced into half rings. Dumplings have the same beige and green skin, but are short and squat and do better cut into wedges.

Zucchini and Yellow Squash—Cut in rounds or diagonals and cook very lightly.

Steamed or parboiled vegetables are a staple of component cooking. Here are a few of the things you can do with them:

1. Add to tossed salads
2. Mix together and add dressing and make a marinated vegetable salad. For variety add things like olives, avocado, jalapeno peppers, cheese cubes, crumbled feta or blue cheese, turkey, ham, chicken, tuna or salmon, sautéed tempeh cubes, etc.
3. Stir-fry chicken, fish, tempeh or meat with seasoning and add vegetables.
4. Cook several vegetables a little bit longer until soft, then purée and season with some herbs and make a quick vegetable soup. Use the original, mineral rich cooking water as your stock if you still have it.

Otherwise use water or a purchased vegetable or chicken stock.

5.   Arrange on a platter and serve with a dip for an hors d'oeuvre that will be very popular.

6.   Eat as-is for snacks, adding some kind of protein.

Thaw Ahead of Time

Take meat, chicken, fish, or frozen entrees and soups out of the freezer several days ahead of time so they can thaw in the refrigerator. If you just take a few minutes to think about what your week will be like, you can begin to develop a habit that will save you from the "just got home from work and there's nothing but cereal to eat" blues. Most items will thaw in your refrigerator in two to three days, depending on their density. A whole chicken, for example, will take longer than a single piece of steak. Here are some other tips for thawing:

• Place meat in some kind of container to catch drips as meat thaws.

• Soups, stews, and sauces can be more quickly thawed by placing entire container in a pan of hot water. Change water as it cools. When food is thawed enough to remove from container, you can usually heat it covered, on a very low temperature. You must keep heat low enough so the liquid released does not evaporate before the solids start to thaw.

Heat Deflectors

A handy kitchen item for cooking "thick" items like stews and oatmeal without scorching them is a *heat deflector.* You can find them in kitchen stores and often in hardware stores that sell kitchen items. A heat deflector looks like two pie pans with holes in them, sealed together, with a handle coming out on one side. Placed between the pan and the burner, the holes allow heat to flow through but keep the pan from direct contact with the burner. A heat deflector can save you from ruining both pots and food!

- If you didn't get something out of the freezer in time, this trick that I learned twenty years ago as a Tupperware dealer works well for steaks, chops, or a pound of ground meat. Bring an inch of water to a boil in a pan and place a steaming basket in it. Turn off the heat, place the wrapped, frozen item in the steamer, cover, and let it sit for 10 to 15 minutes. If the item is still partially frozen, repeat the process. Each time, be sure to turn off the heat as soon as the water boils or the food will cook on the outside. This method will usually get something thawed enough to cook in about 20 minutes.

PLAN A COOKING SESSION

I encourage my clients and students to set aside about three hours once a week to do some food preparation for the week. If you can do this, you will find that during the week your meal preparation time will be reduced to reheating and broiling a piece of fish or quickly cooking a vegetable or two. If you can stock your refrigerator with made-ahead meals, it won't take you any longer to make a healthy, fresh-food meal than it would to drive the kids through a fast food joint or to heat up something equally devoid of nutrition.

"IT'S NOT WORTH IT TO COOK ONLY FOR ME"

If this is your refrain, may I suggest you think about the message you are giving yourself each time you repeat this statement? "I am not worth it," "My health is not important," "It is only worth cooking if there is someone else to cook for." Is this really what you mean to be saying to yourself? More important, is this how you want to treat yourself? Of course it's important to cook for you, even if you are alone. Your health is no less valuable if you are on your own than if you are part of a couple or a family. In fact, one could argue it's even more important, since most single people need to rely on themselves more than people who are coupled.

Oftentimes I think what underlies a reluctance to cook for oneself is that eating alone for many people can underscore a feeling of loneliness. If this is true for you, or if you simply feel like it's too much work to cook for yourself, try teaming up with a friend for cooking sessions. Or find a friend or friends who would be interested in trading some of what they made for some of what you made. It's a great way to try things you might otherwise not have made, it cuts down on the work, and it helps create a support system for eating more healthfully.

CHAPTER NINE

SOMEBODY TELL ME WHAT TO DO!

O ften people have the mistaken belief that eating for health is boring or at the very least, that one would have to be wealthy enough to hire a personal chef to make it interesting. Nothing could be further from the truth. Eating great food is simply a matter of developing some new habits, including the habit of putting some thought into what you're going to eat.

But if you don't cook much, don't have time to cook, or don't like to cook, just the task of thinking up what to have that you haven't had ten times in the last two weeks can be daunting. So I've included forty **menu ideas** to help you get started—twenty for lunches and twenty for dinners. All of the items more complicated than a hard-boiled egg or a piece of fruit are bolded and are included in the cookbook section. If you are following a specific plan (outlined in Chapter Three), you will want to pick menus that provide an appropriate amount of carbohydrate for your needs. If you worked with the carbohydrate portion exercise on page 88, it will probably be fairly easy for you to evaluate any menu. And, after a while, you'll find you can gauge a meal without having to do all the calculating. *All* meal plans as well as recipes in the cookbook are ideal for the Fit and Healthy Plan or anyone who simply wants to stay healthy. If you are following either the Mood-Stabilizing Plan or the Healing Plan, some recipes/menus may have to wait until your health improves. However, because each recipe includes carbohydrate counts, you can easily figure out if a given menu or recipe is for you.

For those of you who say, "If somebody would just tell me what to buy and what to do with it, I'd do it," look at the two **action plans.** The purpose of the action plan is to take you step by step through shopping and cooking for five days. By following an action plan, you can learn a little bit about organizing yourself to shop for and cook several recipes simultaneously. It will also let you experience how planning ahead and setting aside a block of time to cook once a week can make healthy eating far less time-consuming than you think. You may be slow at first if you don't cook much, but that will change over time. Getting the hang of cooking for a week at a time is a big commitment, but one that will pay off tremendously in terms of your health. If the idea seems overwhelming or unappealing, I encourage you to simply read through the action plans in this chapter, then let it go for now. It could be something you grow more comfortable with over time.

Finally, look over *Presto! Change-o!* for ideas on how to become a quick-change artist in the kitchen. Start with one recipe or basic food and see how many different meals you can make from that item. One of the great things about "component" cooking is that it lends itself to creativity and variety.

MENU IDEAS - LUNCHES

Hummus (prepared) Sprouted grain bread Alfalfa sprouts Avocado, cucumber	**Turkey Toss** on shredded romaine lettuce Orange	**Gimme Five Chef's Salad** with **Mustard Apple Vinaigrette**	**Quick Turkey Chili** Small fruit salad with plain low-fat yogurt
Tuna Waldorf Salad w/lettuce and alfalfa sprouts Steamed broccoli	**Tempeh Salad** Celery sticks Apple slices	**Mediterranean Meatloaf** **Sweet 'n' Sour 3-Bean Salad**	**Marinated Vegetable Salad** w/chicken and shredded cheese Orange

MENU IDEAS - LUNCHES *(continued)*

Cream of Asparagus Soup Egg salad Celery and red pepper pieces Kiwi Fruit	Lentil Soup (canned) w/ cooked **kale** and turkey dog (sliced and cooked into soup) **Banana Screams**	**Herb-Roasted Turkey Breast** **Curried Cauliflower Soup** **Hummus** Cut-up red pepper, baby carrots, and cucumber	**Bacon, Lettuce, and Tomato Salad with Smoked Mozzarella** Strawberries
Romaine Roll-Ups **Quinoa Tabouli with Feta Cheese** Cherry tomatoes	Cold Chicken **Jicama Orange Salad** **Carob Fudgie**	Egg salad on bed of alfalfa sprouts Steamed asparagus 100% rye crackers	**Rocky's Mama's Turkey Meatloaf** **Red Garnet Yam** slices Tossed salad/dressing
Simple Chicken Salad Cucumber, peppers, & cherry tomatoes Strawberries	**Judy's Yogurt Sundae** with chopped, toasted almonds	**String Cheese Roll-Ups** **Firecracker Slaw** **Banana Jewels**	Tuna fish salad Cut-up peppers and celery sticks Peach or nectarine

Items in **bold** have recipes included in Cookbook section

MENU IDEAS - DINNERS

Spicy Meatball Mambo **Faux Mashed Potatoes**	**Italian Sausage, Cabbage, and Kraut** Green beans **Apricot Nut Rolls**	**Chicken and Chickpea Stir-Fry** Steamed zucchini	**Salmon Cakes with Horseradish Sauce** **Kale** **Banana Screams**
Tuna-Stuffed Red Pepper Boats **Marinated Vegetable Salad** **Carob Fudgie**	**Quick Thai Chicken** **Brown and Wild Rice** Steamed broccoli	**Ginger Salmon** Salad/dressing **Roasted Curried Sweet Potato**	**Cajun Fish** **Roasted Root Veggies** Steamed broccoli with flaxseed oil
Chicken or Tempeh Fajitas Avocado Low-fat sour cream Tossed salad/dressing	**Cabbage Lasagna** Tossed salad/dressing	**Herb-Roasted Turkey Breast** **Creamy Carrot and Parsnip** Salad with **Mustard Apple Vinaigrette**	**Portuguese Kale and Sausage Soup** with Parmesan Tossed salad/dressing Apple

MENU IDEAS - DINNERS *(continued)*

Turkey Chili Salad with avocado Steamed broccoli	**Indian Meatballs with Yogurt-Cilantro Sauce** **Brown and Wild Rice** Tossed salad/dressing	**Scrod with Ginger Pesto** Parboiled cauliflower **Creamy Carrot and Parsnip**	**Rocky's Mama's Turkey Meatloaf** Steamed green beans **Faux Mashed Potatoes**
BBQ Chicken Steamed Cabbage with flaxseed oil **Berry Delicious Sorbet**	Turkey Burger (from freezer) **Lentil Rice Loaf** **Cucumber Yogurt Salad**	**Crispy Sesame Turkey** Collards Steamed delicata squash	**Glazed Pork and Apple Sauté** Steamed cabbage **Chocolate Mousse**

Items in **bold** have recipes included in the Cookbook section

ACTION PLANS

For my busy weeks, I have always found it easiest to cook ahead on the weekend for the week, and then simply reheat or recombine as I pull together meals during the week. Doing this takes some time to plan and organize and, truth be told, it's not something I can manage to do all the time. When I can, however, it makes my workweek so much easier, not to mention tastier! To do this, you need to think about what to make, how you can use foods in different ways throughout the week, what you need to buy to execute your plan, and in what order you can cook things to be most efficient. A lot of this just comes with experience in the kitchen.

I first created action plans for clients who wanted to change how they were eating but didn't have the time in their lives to do all the thinking and planning involved. If you're not an experienced cook, these two action plans will give you an idea of how to go from idea through execution. Even if you are an experienced cook, you probably do not typically cook a week of meals at one time, and you may find these plans helpful. Each action plan will show you how to coordinate and time the preparation of about a week's worth of food so you can use your kitchen time most efficiently.

I always suggest to my clients that they initially take two to three weeks to implement an action plan, so as not to become overwhelmed. Some people like to team up with a friend, cook together, and share the food. This can be a great way to get and give support for changing your eating habits, especially if you live alone or live with someone who doesn't share your commitment to change.

I've broken the first action plan into two stages: Getting Your Feet Wet and Full-Tilt Boogie. In stage one you will be preparing a few basics to have on hand, like salad dressings, marinades that can be used for meat, fish, chicken, or tempeh, and cut-up raw veggies. These are components that will serve as a base for healthy eating and will allow you to put together some easy meals during the week. You can feel free to stay at stage one for as long as you want to.

Stage two, Full-Tilt Boogie, will take you through all the above, plus parboiled veggies and several entrees that will carry you through your week with minimal additional time in the kitchen. You will learn the art of following several recipes at once, making use of all the spaces of time when one pot is simmering or something else is baking. To save you time, a shopping list for each action plan is also included.

Both of these action plans are suitable for those following any of the three plans outlined in Chapter Three. Those following either the Mood-Stabilizing Plan or the Fit and Healthy Plan can add more healthy carbohydrates according to their needs. After the action plans I have included a meal-planning worksheet to help you continue planning for healthy meals on your own.

Action Plan #1

Here's what you'll be making. I suggest using those sticky paper flags to mark these recipes in the cookbook so you can locate them easily as you cook.

Garden Gaspacho (p. 278)
Nutrition Magician's 4-Bean Salad (p. 313)
Chicken for a Week (p. 316)
Herb-Roasted Turkey Breast (p. 317)
Cut-up Raw Veggies (Peppers, Scallions, Cherry Tomatoes, Celery)
Parboiled Veggies (Broccoli, Carrots, Summer Squash, String Beans) (p.195)
Essential Herb Vinaigrette (p. 262)
Asian Marinade (p. 268)

The menu below shows the meals you can easily pull together throughout the week with the above components. Refer to the page number beside the recipe for instructions on completing that meal. The italicized items are not included in the action plan instructions—these are items you can purchase to fill out your week's menu. They are, however, included on the shopping list.

	Monday	Tuesday	Wednesday
lunch	Tuna Waldorf Salad (p. 354) Raw veggies	Gaspacho *String cheese* *Deli turkey* *Hummus* *Crackers (optional)*	Cold Asian Salmon Nutrition Magician 4-Bean Salad
dinner	Gaspacho Broccoli sautéed in olive oil and garlic	Broiled Asian Salmon with mixed veggies	Chicken Fajitas with *avocado, salsa, and sour cream* (p. 323)

	Thursday	Friday
lunch	*Deli turkey* *Baba ghanouj* *Crackers* *Raw veggies*	Herb-Roasted Turkey Nutrition Magician 4-Bean Salad
dinner	Stir-fry veggies and chicken with **Asian Marinade** (p. 268)	Spanish Meatballs (p. 278, bottom) Salad with avocado and raisins

Getting Your Feet Wet

1. Read over the entire action plan and the recipes listed at the beginning of the action plan, above the menu box. It looks like a lot, but all of the recipes are quick and easy to put together. You will only be doing a few of these in this first stage anyway, so don't panic! (Don't forget the "quick combos" section on page 192 for easy ideas to fill out your menu.)

2. Buy all the staple ingredients—spices, canned goods, oils, vinegars, and any nonperishable items. Buy extras of things used on the quick combo list that you're likely to use regularly, like tuna fish or canned chili.

3. Buy the vegetables on your shopping list marked with an "R." The "R" stands for raw—these items will be cut up for your in-house salad bar. If there is a number after the "R," it indicates that vegetable is also used in a cooked recipe. Buy only the smaller quantity noted after the "R" for your cut-up raw veggies (of course, buy a larger quantity if you think you'll use them). If you have time, rinse, wash, and cut up veggies before putting away to have them on hand. Cucumbers dry out, so don't do them ahead; and remember, peppers and scallions keep best in glass jars or containers. Lettuce that is not purchased prewashed can be washed, dried, wrapped in paper toweling, and stored in a plastic bag. Only do enough for two or three days or the lettuce will get slimy and "rusty."

4. Make the Essential Herb Vinaigrette and the Asian Marinade to have on hand—they keep forever in glass jars in fridge.

5. Do just this much until you're comfortable with it, then add a few new things—maybe some parboiled veggies, maybe the Chicken for a Week recipe. Then, when you're ready for another leap, proceed to stage two.

Full-Tilt Boogie

This is the week you feel ready to tackle the cooking. Shop for all the perishable items on the shopping list, preferably close to the day you're going to cook. You may find you are buying more food than you have in the past, especially vegetables. There will also be new staples that are gradually going to fill your pantry as you try new recipes. As fresh, whole foods become a larger part of your diet, your refrigerator may be a lot fuller, as these foods aren't nearly as compact as highly processed foods.

If you don't plan to cook within two to three days of shopping, freeze meat and poultry. Fish is best used on the day it's purchased, or at the latest, the next day. By day three it has a smell that gives it its bad reputation! Be aware that frozen items will take two to three days to thaw in refrigerator (two days for fish, ground meat, chops, steaks, or boneless chicken, three days for most thicker cuts of meat, whole chickens, and bone-in, cut-up poultry). If you have time, prep all the raw veggies, as in week one, before putting away. Rinse any other fresh veggies that will be used in recipes so they're ready to chop on the day you're going to be cooking. This can also be done at cooking time; it's up to you when you find it most efficient to do. When Cooking Day arrives, read over your recipes again. You may find it easiest to make copies of the recipes you'll be using so you can lay them all out while you cook.

How to Proceed in the Kitchen

1. Start Chicken for a Week and note the time you start it cooking. While chickens are stewing for the first hour, prepare the Herb-Roasted Turkey Breast and get it in the oven. Remember to turn oven temperature down for the turkey breast after 15 minutes. Setting a timer will allow you to let go of remembering this detail.

2. Cut up the veggies you will be parboiling (broccoli, summer squash, 2 large carrots, and 1 lb string beans.) Parboil for 1 to 1½ minutes each, rinse under cold water, and store in one or separate containers as desired. Put string beans aside for Nutrition Magician's 4-Bean Salad. Did you remember to turn the oven temperature down on the turkey breast? (If you are not sure about parboiling, refer to pages 195, 196.)

3. When an hour has passed on stewing the chickens, it's time to take them out of the stock and allow them to cool in a bowl for deboning. Save stock in the pot on stove with no heat under it.

4. Now follow the recipe for the Nutrition Magician's 4-Bean Salad. If you weren't able to find cans of mixed salad beans and bought individual cans of each kind, measure out the amount for the recipe and store the rest in a container for another use. (Look in Presto! Change-o! for hints on how to use them.)

5. Remove the turkey breast from oven when cooking time is up. Let it cool in its pan. The chickens should be cool enough by now to debone. Pull off meat, discard the skin, store chicken in containers and freeze anything you think you won't use in three or four days. Put the bones back in the stock, turn heat back on under pot, and simmer another hour.

6. Make the Gaspacho recipe.

SHOPPING LIST FOR ACTION PLAN #1

Perishables
2 bags prewashed Lettuce (R)
1 pound Green Beans
2 Green Peppers (R)-1
1 head Broccoli
3-4 colored Peppers (R)-2
2 Green Chilies (not Jalapeno)
Large Red Onion
2-3 Sweet White Onions
Garlic (should be a staple)
Large Cucumber or
   3-4 Pickling Cucumbers (R)
Avocado
8 ounces sliced Mushrooms
Celery (R)
1 pound Baby Carrots (R)
3 large Carrots
2 Yellow Summer Squash
Granny Smith or tart Apple
1 Lemon
4-inch piece of Ginger Root
2 pints Grape Tomatoes (R)
1 bunch Green Onions (R)
Small bunch fresh Basil–optional
2½-3 pounds Boneless Turkey Breast
2 Fryer Chickens
1 pound Salmon
½-1 pound deli-sliced Turkey, nitrate-
   and sugar/honey-free
1 pound Ground Sirloin or
   lean Ground Beef

Prepared Foods
Baba Ghanouj
Hummus

Nonperishables
Apricot fruit-only spread
Stevia Liquid
Bay Leaves
Chili Powder
Cinnamon, Cumin, Marjoram
Cloves, Black Peppercorns
Red Pepper Flakes
Sage, Thyme
Tamari
Olive Oil
Sesame Oil
Balsamic or Red Wine Vinegar
Cider Vinegar
Spectrum® Lite Mayonnaise
2 cans Tuna, water-packed
28-ounce can Whole Tomatoes
1 can Westbrae® Salad Beans
1 jar Salsa

Dairy/Eggs
Plain low-fat Yogurt
Low-fat Sour Cream
String Cheese
1 dozen Eggs

Frozen
Orange Juice Concentrate
Sprouted Grain Bread

7. Cut the turkey breast in half when cool. Wrap and freeze half, then wrap and refrigerate the other half (unless, of course, you are serving enough mouths that you need the whole breast at one meal).

8. Strain the chicken stock and discard the bones. Put the stock in containers and refrigerate overnight. Next day, skim off the fat. Divide soup into whatever portions suit you and freeze whatever you won't be using. (No recipe this week calls for chicken stock, so unless you want some for a snack or have another use in mind, you can freeze it for later use.)

9. Good job! Pat yourself on the back for a job well done.

Congratulations! You now have all the components to make the Chicken Fajitas, Asian Marinated Salmon, Chicken and Vegetable Stir-Fry, Turkey Waldorf Salad, and Spanish Meatballs. Each can be assembled and cooked in twenty minutes or less on the day that you want them. All of the other menus can also be assembled quite quickly from the food you have prepared along with the prepared foods that were on the list. Make sure to thaw salmon in advance if it is frozen. Remember, if a recipe calls for an ingredient in its raw state and you are starting with already cooked items (such as with the chicken fajitas), you will shorten the cooking time so that foods are reheated and not overcooked.

Action Plan #2

This week's menu has more things that you will be putting together just before you want to eat them, but all meals should still come together in twenty minutes or less if you've done the preparations ahead of time. Don't forget to flag the recipes for easy reference.

Lemon Rosemary Chicken (p. 330)
Herb-Roasted Turkey Breast (p. 317)
Cut-up Raw Veggies (Red and Green Peppers, Scallions, Cucumber, Cherry Tomatoes, Celery, Mushrooms, Snow Peas, Onion, Lettuce,)
Parboiled Veggies (Broccoli, Carrots, Cauliflower, Green Beans)
Turkey Bacon
Nutrition Magician's Fudge (p. 370)

Mustard Apple Vinaigrette (p. 265)
Essential Herb Vinaigrette (p. 262)

Below are the meals you can easily put together throughout the week with the above components. Refer to the page number beside the recipe for instructions on completing that meal. Again, the italicized items are purchased ready-to-eat and are included on your shopping list.

	Monday	Tuesday	Wednesday
lunch	Bacon, Lettuce, and Tomato Salad (p. 284) Blueberries w/ plain low-fat yogurt and 2 tsp. fruit-only blueberry jam	Gimme Five Chef's Salad (p. 280) 100% rye crackers	Lemon Rosemary Chicken Marinated Vegetable Salad (p. 286)
dinner	Lemon Rosemary Chicken Sautéed broccoli and cauliflower in olive oil and garlic Baked Yam Slices (p. 303)	Turkey Toss (p. 322) Green beans Nutrition Magician's Fudge (p. 370)	Tuna in Red Pepper Boats (p. 355) Strawberries w/ low-fat sour cream

	Thursday	Friday
lunch	Deli Ham String Cheese Roll-Ups Cut-up raw veggies Nutrition Magician's Fudge (p. 370)	Turkey Toss Orange
dinner	Crispy Sesame Fingers (p. 324) Collard greens (p. 290) Marinated Vegetable Salad	Veggie Stir-Fry w/ Shrimp (p. 293) Nutrition Magician's Fudge (p. 370)

As with action plan #1, do this at your own pace, making a limited number of recipes until (and only if) you feel comfortable and ready to try the whole menu. Before you begin, read over each recipe listed above the menu box, as well as How to Proceed in the Kitchen below. I assume you have done your shopping already.

How to Proceed in the Kitchen

1. The Lemon Rosemary Chicken can marinate from 2 to 8 hours, so get it set up ahead of time.
2. Prepare the Herb-Roasted Turkey Breast and put in the oven; don't forget to set a timer for 15 minutes so you'll remember to turn the temperature down.
3. Scrub 2 or 3 yams, wrap each in foil, place on a cookie sheet or in shallow pan, and place in oven with turkey.
4. Fry the turkey bacon and drain on a paper towel. When cool, break into pieces and store in small container in refrigerator. (If you are going to be assembling the BLT Salad during this session, don't bother with the container.)
5. While bacon cooks, begin washing all the vegetables for the Gimme Five Chef's Salad and the BLT Salad. This includes 1 pint cherry or grape tomatoes, 7 cups lettuce, 3 cups mixed greens, a handful of baby carrots or 1 large carrot, and a green pepper.
6. If salads will be used in next few days, cut up the veggies and assemble the salads without dressing and store each in an airtight container. Otherwise store cut-up items separately. Wrap lettuce in paper towel and store in plastic bags, using a separate bag for each salad. Other veggies may be stored in glass jars or well-sealed plastic bags. Don't chop up cucumber or slice cherry tomatoes yet if you aren't assembling the salads.
7. When the turkey breast is done, take it out and allow cooling in the pan. Turn the oven up again to 350° and bake the Lemon Rosemary Chicken. While the oven is open, give your yams a squeeze. If they are soft, take them out, if not, continue cooking along with the chicken. Set a timer for the chicken for 25 minutes, 20 minutes if using boneless chicken. Remove chicken when your timer goes off.

Now bear with me on these next couple steps. Doing it won't be nearly as complicated as reading through it! The gist of it is you have a big pile of vegetables. They'll be used for your Cut-up Raw Veggies, the Marinated

Vegetable Salad, and the Veggie Stir-Fry with Shrimp. Some will need to be parboiled and some left raw.

8. Wash all the vegetables for the Marinated Vegetable Salad and the Veggie Stir-Fry with Shrimp. This includes 2 heads of broccoli, cauliflower, 1 red and 2 green peppers, 1 lb carrots, 1 pint cherry or grape tomatoes, snow peas, and cucumber. Rinse and drain the mung bean sprouts, then put them in a plastic bag until you're ready to make the stir-fry.

9. Cut for parboiling one head of broccoli and the cauliflower for the Marinated Vegetable Salad. You can also cut for parboiling the second head of broccoli and ½ of the carrots you just washed to make the Stir-Fry Veggie and Shrimp dish go together faster during the week. Other vegetables to cut up for the stir-fry (but left raw for now) include the onions and a red and green pepper. Store the onions and the two peppers in separate bags, as they will be added at different times in the stir-fry.

10. Parboil the broccoli, cauliflower, and carrots from step 9. When you have a moment, give your yams a squeeze and see if they are done yet. They probably are, so take them out, cool, and then refrigerate.

11. For the marinated vegetable salad, cut up into a bowl and leave raw the other ½ of the carrots, a green pepper, 1 cucumber, and 1 pint of the cherry tomatoes. You will add the dressing a day before or the morning before you want to eat it. (Remember, if you bought olives, throw those in too.)

12. Make the Mustard Apple Vinaigrette for the Turkey Toss and the Essential Herb Vinaigrette (unless you have some left over) for the BLT, Chef's, and Marinated Vegetable Salads.

13. Make Nutrition Magician's Fudge. Refrigerate.

14. Wrap the cooled turkey breast and refrigerate, freezing part of it if desired. Do the same with the baked chicken.

15. You're done! I know it was a lot of work, but now you are set for the week. All your meals throughout the week can be assembled in ten to twenty minutes.

SHOPPING LIST FOR ACTION PLAN #2

Perishables

2 heads Romaine Lettuce (R)
3 cups Mixed Salad Greens (R)
2 pints Cherry or Grape Tomatoes (R)
1 pound Green Beans
2 pounds Baby or Large Carrots (R)-1lb
1 bunch Collard Greens
2 Cucumbers (R)-1
3 Sweet Red Peppers
5 Green Peppers (R)-2
Celery (R)
Scallions (need 2 each)
2 heads Broccoli
1 Cauliflower
1 medium Onion, white or yellow
1 small Red Onion
½ pound Snow Peas (or Sugar Snaps)
3 cups Mung Bean Sprouts
1 Avocado
4-inch piece Ginger Root
Garlic
2-3 Yams
3 Lemons
1 small Apple
1 pint or quart Strawberries
1 pint Blueberries
2-4 Naval Oranges

8- to 12-ounce package
   Turkey Bacon (chemical-free)
½ pound lean, deli-style Ham
   (chemical-free)
2½-3 pounds Boneless Turkey Breast
1 pound Turkey Tenderloins
1 cut-up Fryer Chicken
1 pound Shrimp

Nonperishables

Dill Pickle Relish
Balsamic or Red Wine Vinegar
Cider Vinegar
Olive Oil
Flaxseed Oil
Sesame Oil
Canola Mayonnaise
Olives (optional for Marinated
   Vegetable Salad)
Tamari
Dijon Mustard
Stevia Liquid
Blueberry Fruit-Only Jam
100 percent Rye Crackers
Almonds (need 2 T)
Sesame Seeds (need ¾ cup)
Dill Weed
Sage
Thyme
Marjoram
Black Pepper
Onion Flakes (need ¾ cup)
Rosemary
Basil
Oregano

Dairy/Eggs

½ pound Smoked Mozzarella
String Cheese
Eggs (need 1)
Plain low-fat Yogurt

MENU-PLANNING WORKSHEET

Recipes for Week

The list is designed to match the way most grocery stores in the United States are organized, with all the fresh, whole foods around the outside perimeter of the store. Pick up frozen items last to prevent thawing before you arrive home. If you set up your own shopping list like this, you will spend less time shopping and eliminate the problem of forgetting something on your list.

1. _____

2. _____

3. _____

4. _____

5. _____

Shopping List:

Produce

Staples (check to see if on hand)

Meat/Fish/Poultry

Dairy

Prepared Foods

Frozen

PRESTO! CHANGE-O!

If you've read through the **Action Plans** (p. 204) and **Component Cooking** (p. 193) you probably have a good idea how you can make a few basic items and turn them into various meals in the days that follow. Below are several examples of ways you can transform basic components into other dishes. Becoming a quick-change artist in the kitchen will keep you from being bored and will help cut down on spoiled and wasted food.

Start with	Turn into
Chicken for a Week (plus stock)	Chicken Salad
	Chicken Waldorf Salad
	Morning Soup
	Chicken Fajitas
	Veggie Stir-Fry with Chicken
	Marinated Vegetable Salad with Chicken
	Gimme Five Chef's Salad with Chicken
	Romaine Roll-Up
	Cream of Any Vegetable Soup (using stock)
Herb-Roasted Turkey Breast	Turkey Waldorf Salad
	Marinated Vegetable Salad with Turkey
	Gimme Five Chef's Salad with Turkey
	Turkey Toss
Brown and Wild Rice Mix	Lentil and Rice Loaf
	Add Mix to a light soup
	Stir-Fried Veggies and Rice Mix with Scrambled Eggs
Baked Yams	Butterscotch Pudding

Start with	Turn into
Asian Marinade	Use on any poultry, fish, or tempeh Marinated Vegetable Salad Veggie Stir-Fry Sauce
Nutrition Magician's BBQ Sauce	Use on chicken, pork, hamburger, turkey burgers, or tempeh Simmer any kind of meatballs in sauce Heat cold, leftover chicken in sauce
Cooked Beans (legumes)	Add to Marinated Vegetable Salad Baked Beans Mash and make refried beans to go with eggs, burgers, or tempeh
Parboiled Vegetables	Veggie Platter with Dip Marinated Vegetable Salads Quick-Blended Vegetable Soup Veggie Stir-Fry Add to Crustless Quiche Add to omelets Sauté in olive oil and garlic Bake in oven with Parmesan cheese Serve with any dressing Top with toasted nuts
Kale or Collard Greens	Portuguese Sausage and Kale Soup Top with Lemon-Miso Tahini Dressing Sauté and add to omelets Add to any soup

CHAPTER TEN

A LITTLE BITE
OF SOMETHING
SWEET

A healthy nutritional lifestyle does not mean being deprived of sweet treats. With some imagination, creativity, and a few new ingredients, you can whip up some pretty darn good stuff that will go over big with people who may not even realize they're eating something that's really good for them. The Cookbook section will provide you with some recipes; all you need is to accumulate some ingredients and add a willing and adventurous spirit!

A TASTE FOR SWEET OR DRUG ADDICTION?

Humans have a natural affinity for sweet-tasting food. Among other things, there's some physiological and evolutionary basis for this, as we have taste buds that are designed to sense sweet. When early humans hunted and gathered food, the sweet tasting mechanism insured survival. Typically foods with a bitter taste were poisonous; a sweet taste was generally indicative of a safe food. Over time, and with the advent of food manufacturing, this taste for sweet has been inflated to the level of an addiction.

Your body is designed to manufacture glucose at a controlled rate to provide fuel for your brain and muscles. It does this by breaking down more complex food until sugar results. The digestion of more complex food allows a controlled release of this vital substance into the bloodstream, insuring proper balance and function of many interconnected systems. Yet the modern diet of fast food, highly refined bread, pasta, cereal and snack foods, and daily sugar consumption bypasses this controlled system on which your body depends. Instead, we ingest pure sugar or food that too quickly becomes pure sugar.

Your body also manufactures natural opiates in the form of the beta-endorphin. We recognize, without question, that it would be unsafe to encourage people to freely self-administer heroin, codeine, or any other form of pure opiate. The dangers are more alarming because death can so easily and immediately result from an overdose of these drugs. But the effects of constant sugar use are clearly linked to disease and death despite the longer time frame. Shouldn't we be just as concerned with this drug, instead of building an economy on its trade?

ARE UNREFINED SWEETENERS BETTER THAN SUGAR?

Over the past twenty years or so, many books and recipes have advocated substituting less refined sweeteners, such as honey or maple syrup, for white sugar. These authors and cooks believe that such ingredients, by virtue of being less refined, improve the healthfulness of the product. While this approach once seemed reasonable, current awareness of the effects of elevated blood sugar and insulin levels requires us to rethink the situation.

While it is true that these alternative sweeteners have a modicum more of nutrient value, from the standpoint of blood sugar and insulin regulation, which is our chief concern, the body recognizes no difference. These concentrated sugars are damaging to the body because of the extreme effect they have on metabolism in the amounts usually eaten. They throw the body out of balance on many levels. These sweeteners are frequently used in combination with other glucose- and insulin-boosting ingredients (most notably, flour, grains, and high sugar fruits) which only compounds the damaging effects.

What this means is that we have to rethink our concept of dessert or treat. Flour- and sugar-laden baked goods, whole grain flour or not, unrefined sweetener or not, will not serve the interests of health. Fat-free sweets are not healthy either; the lack of fat in these products causes blood-sugar and insulin levels to rise higher than they would if fat were included. And often these items contain more sweetener than their fat-containing cousins to make up for the flavor lost by deleting the fat.

RETHINKING DESSERT

Here are some points to consider when you're thinking about how to fit sweet treats into a balanced, healthy nutritional lifestyle:

1. The sweeter the taste, the more likely the food is to raise blood sugar and insulin levels. This is true for fruits and vegetables as well as sugars and sweeteners.

2. Sweet foods should generally be eaten in small quantities.

3. Sweet foods will be utilized more healthfully if eaten as part of a meal instead of on their own. They are also less likely to trigger cravings for more sweets when eaten this way.

4. The ideal recipe for a sweet treat contains a reasonable balance of protein, fat, and carbohydrate. Or, if the recipe is significantly heavier in carbohydrate, make sure the food is eaten with protein.

5. The fact that a sweet food has few or no calories does not guarantee it will not trigger the release of insulin or food cravings. Some noncaloric, natural, and artificial sweeteners trigger the release of insulin in *some* people.

NEW INGREDIENTS

Creating treats that meet the criteria of being balanced in macronutrient (protein, fat, and carbohydrate) composition, easy on blood-sugar and insulin levels, and great tasting will require you to learn about and start using some new ingredients. A few of these will be described below, along with some supplementary information on where and how you may purchase them. Depending on where you live, not all ingredients will be available to you in local retail stores. For each item, I have provided you with an online source from which you can order.

Right now, the concepts of lower- or controlled-carbohydrate eating are trendy. Over the next few years, we will see this trend integrated into mainstream thought about healthy eating, and as we saw with the low-fat trend, more and more companies will bring new products to the marketplace to meet consumer demand. This is already happening online and you can expect to see that carrying over into brick and mortar retail establishments. It will be important for you as the consumer, however, to read ingredient labels and still be on the lookout for use of chemical sweeteners, hydrogenated fats, concentrated soy foods, and other unhealthy ingredients contained within these products.

LOW- OR NO-GLYCEMIC SWEETENERS

There are several low-glycemic or no-glycemic sweeteners on the market that can be substituted for insulin-boosting sweeteners in many recipes. When using these sweeteners you may have to experiment a little to discover how much to use. Some are quite potent and a minute amount will go a long way.

It's important to mention that, for some people, just the taste of sweetness may stimulate insulin to be released, which can then cause food cravings. You will need to monitor your own reactions and make adjustments in your habits if this applies to you. For the people who have this level of sensitivity, sometimes eating only mildly sweet foods and combining them with a meal can lessen this problem. Generally, this reaction indicates a high degree of imbalance and a need for healing. Following the Healing Plan will typically bring the body back into balance.

Stevia

Stevia is an herbal sweetener from a plant native to South America where it has been used for centuries. It has been used commercially for decades in Japan. Stevia is 300 times sweeter than sugar! You can buy it as a liquid extract or in powder form at most health food stores. You may have choices between a clear or brown liquid and between green or white powder. I suggest the clear liquid and/or the white powder for best appearance in your recipes. I typically use the liquid in my recipes because I find it easier to regulate the amount. Many cookbooks that include stevia, however, use the powder.

Stevia is so potent a tiny amount is usually all that's necessary. Too much stevia gives the food or drink a licorice aftertaste. More often than not, the amount you need to produce adequate sweetness will not be enough to give the aftertaste.

REPLACING SUGAR WITH STEVIA			
Amount of Sugar in Recipe	1 Cup	1 Tablespoon	1 teaspoon
Amount of Stevia Powder	1 teaspoon	¼ teaspoon	pinch to $\frac{1}{16}$ teaspoon
Amount of Stevia Liquid	1 teaspoon	6-9 drops	6-9 drops

When following a recipe that uses stevia, I always start with less than the recipe calls for and work up. Everyone's taste for sweet varies; yours will no doubt change over time as your body heals. I have found in most recipes using stevia, I need to adjust down.

Stevia has been approved by the FDA for use as a supplement, but not as a food. Because of this you will find it in health food stores in the supplement section, not, as you might expect, with the sweeteners. If you do not have access to a store that carries stevia, you can look on line at **www.stevia.com** or type "stevia" in the keyword line of a search engine. This will give you a number of commercial sites from which to choose.

Trutina

Trutina is a low-glycemic natural sweetener made from kiwi fruit. It has just less than 5g of carbohydrate per teaspoon, and is 10 times as sweet as sugar measure for measure. This product is available at **www.thermofit.com.**

Sucralose

Sucralose is the generic name for a chemical sweetener that claims no effect on insulin. It has been in use in Canada for many years and has just recently been approved for sale in the US by the FDA. I have some concerns about Sucralose and don't recommend its use at this time. There are no independent studies (meaning studies not conducted by the manufacturer) on human use, and outside experts who have analyzed study data contest many of the manufacturer's claims to its safety. In animal tests, Sucralose has been shown to shrink the thymus gland and stunt the growth of rats.

Sucralose is made by chlorinating sugar molecules. In other words it is a chemical, rather than natural, product. There are many unanswered questions about the potential long-term effects of manipulating the molecular structure in this way. If you would like to read more about the issues relevant to its safety, type "sucralose" into any search engine. Just be aware of whether the article is coming from an industry lobby group or an independent organization with no financial connection to products containing Sucralose. The fact is, we simply don't know that Sucralose is safe, despite its approval by the FDA.

Sucralose is being used in more and more manufactured foods including:

- Baked goods and baking mixes
- Chewing gum
- Confections and frostings
- Fats and oils (salad dressings)
- Fruit and water ices
- Jams and jellies
- Processed fruits and fruit juices
- Sweet sauces, toppings, and syrups
- Beverages and beverage bases
- Coffee and tea
- Dairy product analogs
- Frozen dairy desserts and mixes
- Gelatins, puddings, and fillings
- Milk products
- Sugar substitutes

I urge you to use awareness in experimenting with these sweeteners. Because most of us are so easily addicted to the taste of sweet, it would be easy to keep our taste buds and body craving sweet food. Your health is best served by taming that craving and putting sweet food in its place within a balanced a diet. There is nothing wrong with enjoying the pleasure of a sweet treat. Each person has to determine whether his or her desire for something sweet has the charge of an addictive craving or not. As mentioned earlier, many people find the taste of sweet alone enough to trigger an insulin response from the body, followed by hunger or by sweet/carbohydrate cravings. Also, many people who are trying to lose weight report that frequent use of these sweeteners stalls their progress. Since everyone's body is different you have to watch *your* responses and make appropriate modifications.

IS FOOD ENOUGH OR DO YOU NEED SUPPLEMENTS?

S upplements have become both big business and an accepted part of holistic health care in the last decade. We are constantly bombarded with television and newspaper or magazine items praising or condemning this herb or that vitamin. The Internet is loaded with sites that offer information, recommendations, and products for sale. So how can you go about evaluating whether you should be using supplements and, if so, which ones?

The first issue to discuss, even before we talk about supplements themselves, is how we think about supplements. We live in a "quick-fix" culture; when we have symptom or an illness, most of us think immediately "How can I get rid of this problem?" Now there's certainly nothing wrong with wanting to feel better and be rid of an illness or uncomfortable condition. And sometimes, we need a fast-acting solution so that we are able to go on to address the underlying problem. If your blood pressure is sky high, medication to lower it may be appropriate in the short term until you can work on lifestyle changes to keep it down. Or if you are so depressed that going through the day is difficult, you may benefit from antidepressants so you can find the energy and clarity to make more holistic changes. But is eliminating the symptom *without addressing its underlying cause* really what you want to do? I hope not. In the short term you may feel better, but with respect to your long-term well-being and health, you are not doing yourself any favors.

Many health-conscious individuals avoid taking prescription medications for a health problem, preferring instead to look for a natural herb or supplement to take its place. In some cases, this is just substituting a different substance into the same "quick-fix" thinking. Admittedly, most herbal remedies and supplements are more benign and don't have the levels of toxicity that manufactured pharmaceuticals do. But herbs and supplements are not harmless, and they may only be a marginally better solution if using them helps you to avoid asking the question, "Why does my body need this substance in the first place?" This chapter is meant to help you think more holistically about the use of supplements.

DO YOU HAVE A NEED FOR SUPPLEMENTS?

Before you begin your search for the right supplement, here are some questions to consider:

- Is my diet supplying adequate nutrition?
- Is my body able to absorb and utilize the nutrients it is being given through food?
- Does my present life and lifestyle expose me to stresses that increase my need for certain nutrients?
- Do I have an imbalance in brain or body chemistry that can be corrected or helped with supplements?

To answer some of these questions you may need the help of a qualified health care practitioner. In my experience, holistic and nutritionally aware chiropractors (DC), naturopathic doctors (ND), osteopathic doctors (DO), and some holistically thinking medical doctors (MD) are helpful in looking at the big picture. Although medical schools that train MDs are incorporating more alternative and natural approaches to medicine, often the approach to supplements is still along the lines of "take a pill to cure a symptom." I encourage you to find a practitioner, whatever initials follow his or her name, who has a whole-body, systemic approach.

There are generally four reasons that people choose to take supplements:

1. To eliminate a symptom
2. To correct an underlying imbalance
3. To supplement an adequate diet
4. To supplement an inadequate diet

Let's consider each one.

1. Eliminating a symptom

Sometimes eliminating a symptom with a supplement may be appropriate. For instance, using the very effective herb uva ursi to treat a urinary tract infection or taking the amino acid supplement GABA to reduce anxiety are two examples. However, if these symptoms are either chronic or recurring, merely treating the symptom is not enough. When a symptom is persistent, it is an indication that some imbalance exists within one's body or lifestyle, and continuing to medicate, albeit with a nonpharmaceutical, simply prolongs the imbalance.

2. Correcting an underlying imbalance

Some imbalances in the body may not only produce a set of specific symptoms, but can also cause further imbalance. A very common example is the imbalance in brain chemistry discussed in Chapter Three that leads to depression. Low serotonin and low beta-endorphin levels, a condition a person may have inherited, leads the person to crave sugar and/or refined carbohydrates. Eating these foods leads to blood sugar imbalance, which creates cravings for more of the same foods. The original neurotransmitter imbalances lead to depression and lack of energy, which are then exacerbated by the diet. Depression and lethargy make exercising or being active difficult, which makes it hard for the person to raise his or her beta-endorphin level. A diet high in sugar and carbohydrate brings the brain chemistry further out of balance and is likely to lead to other imbalances, such as obesity, diabetes, hypothyroidism, chronic fatigue, chronic systemic yeast (candida), elevated blood lipids, etc. As you can see, this is a cyclical problem that can bring health into a downward spiral.

In a case such as this, not at all unusual in my practice, if I were to suggest supplements to help eliminate chronic yeast, for example, the person would likely get no relief from their symptoms without eliminating refined carbohydrates and sugar from his or her diet, since those foods feed yeast. With the appropriate dietary change, he or she would likely see a clearing of the yeast, as well as changes in all the other symptoms of imbalance—excess weight, depression, elevated blood lipids, and diabetes, to name a few. In this case, a candida-fighting supplement would be useful in clearing the symptom because the underlying cause of the imbalance was being addressed.

Another very common problem I see in my practice is the problem of adult onset or Type II diabetes. In the very early stages, even before diabetes has been diagnosed, a person may spend years being insulin-resistant, a problem we discussed in Chapter One. Insulin resistance and the diet that leads to it can result in all of the problems from the example above. Suppose this person complains of fatigue to her friend and the friend suggests an herbal supplement that promotes weight loss and also boosts energy. If our insulin-resistant person follows the friend's suggestion and uses this supplement to "cure" her fatigue (also hoping to lose a few pounds), she will create bigger health problems for herself down the road. Herbal weight loss supplements usually contain one or more kinds of stimulants, which although "all natural" have a negative effect on the body. These stimulants trigger the adrenal glands and cause the body to produce an excess of stress hormones, which can interfere with fat metabolism and insulin regulation, and elevate the risk for heart disease. Neither would taking these supplements address the underlying problem of insulin resistance. Picking out only one problem to treat is not likely to lead to a very satisfactory outcome in terms of overall health. This is why the "one symptom, one supplement" (or "one medication") approach is not effective.

Many levels of imbalance may exist in your body—hormones may be out of balance, organs may be improperly functioning, your body may be toxic from pollutants in air, water, food, or the chemicals used in your home or yard. When one treats each symptom independently without assessing the whole picture, the result is often a gradual—or sometimes not-so-gradual— deterioration in health. In our society, unfortunately, we often call this "aging."

3. Supplementing an adequate diet

Let's assume you're in good health, you're in balance, and you eat a diet low in refined carbohydrates, adequate in protein and healthy fat, and containing a large variety of fresh vegetables and moderate amounts of fruit. Your body is able to extract and assimilate the nutrition available from the food you eat. Can you benefit from supplements?

In my opinion, yes, and here's why. First of all, it's good insurance. No one eats a great diet all the time, unless they are extremely motivated and have nothing else to take care of in life. Second, the nutrient composition of food is highly variable. The amount of any nutrient available in a given food is going to depend on soil and growing conditions, time and storage conditions between harvest and when you eat it, cooking method, and other foods eaten in combination with it. If you happen to be using pharmaceutical medication, it may affect your body's ability to utilize some nutrients or change your body's need for a particular nutrient. (Birth control pills, for example, deplete the body of B vitamins.) And, finally, we are subject to many stresses in modern life, which put an increased burden on our body. Time pressure, multitasking, use of technology that exposes us to electromagnetic fields, and exposure to toxins all change the body in ways we're only beginning to measure and understand. These stresses in your life increase your need for biological support.

TAKE TWO APPLES AND CALL ME IN THE MORNING

All of the stress in your life also increases the *oxidative stress* on your body. **Oxidative stress** can be thought of in simple terms as something that causes your body to "rust" from the inside out. Visualize how rust eats away at a car's body. Well, oxidative stress occurs when unstable molecules called **free radicals** nibble away at your cells, compromising their integrity and function. If the cell wall structure is compromised, the cell's insides, including your genetic material, are more vulnerable to bacteria, viruses, and cancer-causing molecules. Stress is what causes the production of unstable, free radicals in your body, even good stress like exercise. But free radicals are even more abundant with bad stress caused by toxins, electromagnetic fields, stored-up emotions, tobacco, drugs, and alcohol, to name a few examples. The group of supplements known as **antioxidants** can neutralize free radicals so the damage to your body is minimized.

4. Supplementing an inadequate diet

This is probably the most common reason people take supplements. The supplement user in this category diet may be relying on supplements to address a symptom rather than to correct an underlying imbalance, or to compensate for a poor diet overall. I don't recommend long-term reliance on supplements to make up for an inadequate diet; obviously you would be far better off making lifestyle changes that would allow you to feed yourself for maximum health and vitality. But I am a realist, and there are circumstances that might prevent you from receiving the care you need to address deeper levels of imbalance, or from eating a nutritionally adequate diet. In these circumstances, using supplements to boost health would generally be a better alternative than not using them.

One note of caution here: If a supplement merely masks a deeper level of imbalance, you risk more serious health consequences if you don't find and resolve the deeper problem. Supplements are no better than pharmaceutical drugs in this respect themselves, although they are likely to be less toxic to the body.

FOOD-BASED VERSUS SYNTHETIC SUPPLEMENTS

Supplements can be divided into two categories: natural, meaning food-based, and synthetic. This can be tricky when selecting supplements because the supplement industry has come to use the term "natural," quite loosely, and something labeled "natural" may not be. For instance, vitamin C occurs naturally in plants, but most vitamin C in the market is synthesized in a laboratory. Another example, vitamin E, also occurs naturally in many foods and is an important antioxidant. Vitamin E has many different forms (called tocopherols) and when present in food is accompanied by many other vitamins, minerals, and phytochemicals. Laboratory-synthesized vitamin E may offer only one kind of tocopherol, without all the other goodies that you get when you eat a whole food containing vitamin E.

Your body does not metabolize a nutrient ingested as a single component the same way it would if that same nutrient were presented in the complex structure of food with all its nutrient relatives. Nutrients are designed by nature to work together within your body. This happens best, of course, when you eat a variety of whole foods on a daily basis. The next best thing is to take supplements that are derived from whole foods. The vitamin C you take in pill form is not the same vitamin C you get when you eat an orange or some broccoli. And it doesn't act the same way in your body. Chiropractor and naturopath Darren Schmidt, a colleague of mine, explains it this way: "The vitamin C molecule is huge. It contains many other elements beside ascorbic acid; in fact, only a tiny amount is ascorbic acid. All those other elements are part of what makes it effective in your body. The vitamin C that you get in a whole-food-based supplement, even though it contains a tiny amount of ascorbic acid, will be far more effective than taking a mega-dose of ascorbic acid as we're accustomed to doing. The whole food supplement will strengthen and nourish many parts of the body, so the whole body functions better."

Products made from whole-food concentrates may contain many things besides the single nutrient we've become so used to purchasing at the health food store. Companies that make whole-food-based supplements pick the food that research has determined will provide the most effective source of that particular vitamin. Many chiropractors, naturopaths, osteopaths, and holistic doctors are knowledgeable about supplementing through the use of whole food-concentrates.

Many synthetic supplements use tablets that contain sugar, wheat, corn, or dairy, all potential allergens for many people. And less conscientious manufacturers may use coatings on their tablets that make them less digestible and absorbable. In some cases, a particular nutrient needs one or more other nutrients to be utilized; a common example of this is calcium, which needs magnesium to be well-absorbed. It's best to educate yourself or work with a knowledgeable holistic health practitioner to get the most out of any supplements you may be using.

HERBS AND HERBAL PREPARATIONS

Herbs have been used medicinally for centuries by medicine men and women, shamans, and all manner of healers. Though natural, herbs—like supplements—can be approached with either the "one symptom-one herb mentality" or with a more holistic mindset.

Herbs, by their very nature, are whole foods. Depending on how they are prepared, and how concentrated the preparation is, they can be used to nourish, balance, and support the body, gradually bringing things into greater balance, or they can have a more immediate effect, much like a drug. Master herbalist and author Susun Weed has written several excellent books that can serve as a reference for healing with herbs. I recommend you start with either *Healing Wise* or *New Menopausal Years*.

Herbs are not without their risks and side effects, although, to be sure, the dangers in most cases are far less than those of prescription drugs. The average fatality rate from herbs is about four deaths per year compared to over 100,000 deaths annually from legal use of prescription drugs. Many herbs are contraindicated for pregnant women. And many can interact with prescription medication, either increasing or counteracting its effect. There are a lot of herbs that have a blood-thinning effect, for example, and can compound the effect of anticoagulant drugs. Some herbs can help protect against the toxic side effects of pharmaceuticals; for instance, the herb milk thistle helps protect the liver from the potential damage of cholesterol-lowering drugs. It is always wise to investigate the potential drug interactions of any herb you're considering taking and to let your health care practitioner know what you are taking. If you have a preference for letting the herb do the job instead of the drug, there are many cases where lab tests can monitor the effectiveness of the herb or can be used to make sure that you are not overshooting the mark.

One good print source I use is a book called *Herb Contraindications and Drug Interactions*, by Francis Brinker, N. D., and there have been several others published recently. If you use herbs, I strongly recommend you to get one as a reference. You can check herb-drug interactions through online sources as well. As this area of investigation is fairly new, there will probably be more sites and updated information available as time goes on.

One of the most comprehensive sites covering herb-drug interactions that I have found is **www.lifebalm.com/drug_herb3.html**. This site has charts organized by herb type. Another site, **www.uspharmacist.com/ NewLook/DisplayArticle.cfm?item_num=566,** contains a very detailed chart organized by medication type that health professionals and health consumers alike can use to assess potential herb-drug interactions. The chart also provides specific symptoms of a harmful interaction, including information for doctors on changes in lab test values that may indicate a problem. Some medical-based sites that offer herb-drug interaction information have a clear bias towards the use of pharmaceuticals; the site above provides information that would allow patient and practitioner to make an informed decision based on science, not politics.

HERBAL TINCTURES

One of the ways to get the most benefit from herbal medicine is to use herbal tinctures. Tinctures are a liquid extract made by covering the plant material with alcohol for about a month. This allows the active plant alkaloids to transfer to the liquid, which is then bottled as the tincture. Tincture drops are added to drinking water.

One of the best sources of carefully made, high-quality tinctures can be found at a one-woman business created and run by herbalist Cathy Hope of New Mexico. Iris Herbal specializes in preparations from high-quality, organically grown and wildcrafted herbs. Wildcrafted herbs are grown in the wild and gathered with respect for both the plants' growing cycles, which affect the herb's potency, and its place in the ecosystem within which it grows. You can learn more about herbs and Iris Herbal at **www.irisherbal.com/index.html** or by calling 1-877-286-2970.

CHOOSING GOOD-QUALITY SUPPLEMENTS

Food-based supplements are available in some health food stores and from many holistic health practitioners and can also be purchased through direct-marketing companies, also known as multilevel marketing companies. Concerning the latter, there is no need to be frightened of buying products from a company that uses this method of marketing. There are some very good companies and products being marketed this way. A company that markets through person-to-person marketing is not any more or less likely than a traditional company to sell an inferior product. You need to do your homework no matter from whom you buy.

One issue concerning herbs and supplements that has received media attention is the issue of standardization, meaning that each batch of a supplement contains what it says it does in the amounts claimed on the label. There is no certain way as of yet to be sure an herbal or supplement product is true to its label claim, as the FDA does not presently regulate the supplement industry in this way. There is a company called Consumer Labs that has recently started conducting tests of selected categories of supplements and nutritional products and makes the results available on their website **www.consumerlab.com**. However, they do not test every brand within a category. The site will allow you to see an overview of the testing results for free and then charges a small annual fee ($17.95 at last check) for access to specific brand information.

The issue of standardization is perhaps more relevant when dealing with synthetically formulated supplements. When taking food-based supplements, remember that any plant is going to vary in its chemical/nutrient composition depending on many factors, not unlike the differences you might find between heads of broccoli grown on two different farms. Food manufacturers or the Department of Agriculture assign nutrient values to food items all the time, but those numbers are only averages. We don't concern ourselves with whether each package of broccoli au gratin has the exact amount of vitamin C that the label specifies, because eating a whole food typically does not put us at risk if it contains more or less of a nutrient. The same is true for supplements based on whole food concentrates. Remember that a nutrient taken in whole food form is generally safer and more effective than a synthetic product. Research studies that try to measure the effectiveness of a single vitamin or nutrient really say nothing about the synergistic effect of that nutrient if it were used in whole food form. It still pays, however, to purchase your herbal or whole-food supplements from companies known to be reputable for their quality products.

EVALUATING HERB OR SUPPLEMENT EFFECTIVENESS

This procedure is useful when you are using an herb or supplement for a specific problem. Supplements that offer overall biological support, such as antioxidants, are intended to be taken continuously.

1. Make sure the herb or supplement you're considering is safe for you.

2. Start at a reasonable, recommended dose; take for one month.

3. If you don't notice any change or notice only minimal change, increase dose for another month.

4. Repeat until you get desired result or reach maximum safe dosage.

5. If effective, maintain three to six months then gradually wean yourself off.

---

6. During next 30 days see how you feel. If you feel better, discontinue supplement. If you notice no change, regimen may no longer be needed.

Overall, I encourage you to seek help from a qualified health practitioner for determining an optimal supplement program for you, in conjunction with a health program that includes nutrition and exercise as its base.

RESOURCES

Chapter 1: The Importance of Blood-Sugar and Insulin Regulation

Eat Wild
Very informative site about the health benefits of meat from grass-fed animals and sources for purchasing.
www.eatwild.com

Chapter 2: Fat Fiction, Lean Fact

Know Your Fats: The Complete Primer for Understanding the Nutrition of Fats, Oils and Cholesterol, Mary K. Enig, Ph.D., Bethesda Press
An excellent book about fats that also critically evaluates the cholesterol-heart disease research, by a leading lipid researcher.
www.bethesdapress.com or **(301) 680-8600**

Weston A. Price Foundation for Wise Traditions in Food, Farming and the Healing Arts
Leading educational organization supporting intelligent nutrition, community-supported agriculture, organic farming, etc.
www.westonaprice.org

Chapter 4: Jumpstarting Your Metabolism

Complete Book of Food Counts, Corinne T. Netzer, Mass Market Paperback
Comprehensive reference book for nutrient analysis.

Sources for user-friendly nutrition software:
www.lifeform.com (PC's)
www.arealinks.net/Cyberdiet (MAC's)

Chapter 5: Something to Drink: More Than an Afterthought

Caffeine Blues, Stephen Cherniske, M.S., Warner Books 1998
A comprehensive summary of caffeine research. Cherniske is a leading
health journalist and gives in-depth information in an easy-to-read style.

Your Body's Many Cries for Water, Global Health Solutions Inc.,
Batmanghelidj, F., M.D.
Not always easy to follow, this is worth reading to gain a greater
appreciation for the importance of water to our health.
See also **www.watercure.com**

Chapter 6: Hormone Balance and Imbalance—The Big Eight

*Screaming to Be Heard: Hormonal Connections Women Suspect and
Doctors Still Ignore,* Elizabeth Lee Vliet, M.D., M. Evans and Company,
Inc. Revised 2000
This book addresses most health issues women face relating to
hormones and will provide any woman the background she needs to be
her own health advocate.

Site with excellent information about thyroid disease:
www.about.com.
Click on the link for health and fitness, then thyroid disease under
"diseases and conditions."

National Women's Health Network
Site of a non-profit research organization for women's health that accepts
no funding from pharmaceutical, tobacco, or medical device manufacturers:
www.womenshealthnetwork.org or **(202) 628-7814**

What Your Doctor May Not Be Telling You about Menopause, John R.
Lee, M.D., Warner Books, 2002
Dr. Lee was one of the first authors to raise the issue of estrogen dominance

and advocate for the use of progesterone cream in dealing with symptoms related to peri-menopause and menopause.
www.johnleemd.com

Source for Progesterone Cream:
Arbonne International, PhytoProlief
www.arbonne.com

The Miracle of Natural Hormones, David Brownstein, M.D., Medical Alternative Press, 1999
An easy-to-read, comprehensive look at the roles and interconnections of the major hormones affecting our health yet often ignored by doctors.
www.drbrownstein.com or **(888) 647-5616**

Healing with Whole Foods, Paul Pitchford, North Atlantic Books, 2001
Pitchford comes from the perspective of Chinese medicine and presents an extremely well-organized resource. Whether or not you understand a lot about Chinese medicine, you can learn a lot about the medicinal properties of food.
www.northatlanticbooks.com or **800-337-BOOK (2665)**

Sites that present worldwide research on the problems related to soy consumption:
www.soyonlineservice.co.nz
www.westonaprice.org

Strong Women Stay Young, Miriam Nelson, Ph.D. with Sarah Wernick, Ph.D., Bantam Books, 2000
In my opinion, the best book for women who are new to strength training and want a way to begin gently, but effectively.

Chapter Seven: Practically Speaking

National Organization Mobilized to Stop Glutamate
Site for anyone concerned with or curious about the problem of MSG sensitivity:
www.nomsg.com or **800-232-8674**

Chapter Ten: A Little Bite of Something Sweet

Sources for low- and no-glycemic sweeteners:
www.stevia.com
www.thermofit.com (for trutina dulcem)

The Stevia Cookbook: Cooking with Nature's Calorie-Free Sweetener, by Ray Sahelian, M.D., and Donna Gates, Penguin Putnam Inc, 1999
Not all recipes in this book are suitable for a controlled-carbohydrate lifestyle, but the book has great information for those unfamiliar with stevia and how to use it.

Appendix 1: Is Food Enough or Do You Need Supplements?

Healing Wise (Wise Woman Herbal Series), Susun S. Weed, Ash Tree Publishing, 1989

New Menopausal Years, The Wise Woman Way: Alternative Approaches for Women 30-90 (Wise Woman Herbal Series, Book 5), Susun S. Weed, Ash Tree Publishing, 2000
Weed is one of the more influential voices for women in the use of herbs and healing. *New Menopausal Years* is a great reference to have on hand long before the time comes.

Sites with good information about herb-drug interactions:
www.lifebalm.com

U.S. Pharmacist
www.uspharmacist.com/NewLook/DisplayArticle.cfm?item_num=566
(U.S. Pharmacist, Vol 25:8, *A Review of Herb-Drug Interactions: Documented and Theoretical)*

Iris Herbal
Great source for herbal products from leading herbalist Cathy Hope:
www.irisherbal.com/index.html or **1-877-286-2970**

Watchdog site reporting on testing for quality supplements:
www.consumerlab.com

THE
TAKE TWO
APPLES
COOKBOOK

BREAKFASTS

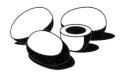

PROTEIN SMOOTHIE

Serves 1

This basic smoothie can be varied in ways limited only by your imagination. Whey protein is utilized quickly by your body, so a smoothie alone for breakfast may only last you about 2 hours. It's a great breakfast for those who otherwise wouldn't eat anything. It also makes a great snack, and kids love them.

3 rounded tablespoons (1 scoop) **Whey Protein Powder***
    (vanilla, strawberry, or chocolate)
½ cup **Water** (to taste) or **Milk** or some combination of both
4 **Ice Cubes**
⅓ frozen medium **Banana** or 5 frozen **Strawberries** or ½ **Apple** (optional)
1 tablespoon **Flaxseed Oil** or **Walnut Oil** or 2 tablespoons **Coconut Milk**
Flavored Extract of Choice
    coffee, vanilla, maple, coconut…etc. (optional)
Spice of Choice
    cinnamon, nutmeg, cardamom (optional)

1. Place all ingredients in a blender. (It helps to crush the ice cubes with a hammer first.)

2. Blend on high until texture is smooth.

1 serving =
With 2% milk, fruit: 314 kcal; 27g protein; 18g carbohydrate; 18g fat (1g saturated)
With water, fruit: 253 kcal; 23g protein; 12g carbohydrate; 15.7g unsaturated fat
With water, no fruit: 218 kcal; 23g protein; 3g carbohydrate; 15.5g unsaturated fat

Note: If you are following a plan in which fruit is limited, this shake tastes great without fruit as well. I sometimes use 1 tablespoon flax meal instead of the oil to give the shake extra thickness if I don't use fruit.

---

*I recommend buying chocolate, vanilla, or strawberry whey protein powder from Jay Robb Enterprises. This is the only brand I know of that has no sugars or artificial sweeteners and still tastes great! JRE uses stevia, a very sweet herb with no effect on blood glucose levels. You can purchase in 1- or 2-pound cans.
1-800 862-8763 or **www.jayrobb.com**

If you are allergic to dairy or are lactose-intolerant, you may substitute Jay Robb Egg White Protein Powder. The Egg White Protein Powder does not have as much stevia, and you will need to add stevia to taste. Many people who are lactose-intolerant can use whey protein powder because most of the lactose is removed.

Variations:
Follow the basic formula with the following changes:

Lemon Blueberry Cheesecake—Vanilla Whey Powder, ½ cup frozen Blueberries, ⅓ teaspoon Lemon Extract

Mocha Almond Fudge—Chocolate Whey, 1 tablespoon Almond Butter and omit Flax Oil, ½ teaspoon Coffee Extract

Chocolate Mint—Chocolate Whey, ½ teaspoon Peppermint Extract (or to taste)

Butterscotch Kiss—Vanilla Whey, 1 tablespoon Almond Butter and omit Flax Oil, ½ teaspoon Butterscotch Extract

Strawberry Tropical Treat—Strawberry or Vanilla Whey, ½ cup frozen Strawberries, ½ teaspoon Coconut Extract

---

EGG CREPES À LA BOYDSTUN
Serves 2

Sally Boydstun makes the best chocolate truffles I know and is also a most creative, low-carbohydrate cook. This just goes to show that life isn't black and white. Sally came up with this nifty breakfast or brunch idea. I have adapted her recipe and added some fillings. The recipe serves one or two depending on filling and rest of meal.

1 whole **Egg**
2 **Egg Whites**
Salt, Pepper, and Herbs and/or Spices of choice
Olive Oil

1. Whip the eggs and whites together. Heat a small (about 6½ inch) omelet pan. This is a small frying pan with curved sides. Using a mister, add tiny bit of oil or spray, just enough to coat pan. With heat on medium, pour scant ¼ cup well-mixed egg mixture into pan. Allow to cook until bottom is set, about 15 seconds.

2. Use a metal turner and gently go around the edge of crepe, lifting to make sure it isn't sticking. Then gently flip crepe over. Cook for 8-10 seconds more and gently turn onto platter.

3. Make remaining "crepes." Fill with any of the fillings below. Makes 4 crepes.

Blintz
Blend together ½ cup ricotta cheese with 1 teaspoon vanilla extract, stevia drops to taste, and, if desired, cinnamon. Spread 2 tablespoons of filling on each egg crepe and roll up. Optional additions: fruit-only jam, sautéed apple slices, chopped nuts.

Sautéed Veggies
Any combination of veggies that you like in an omelet would go well here. Mushrooms, onions, green or red Bell peppers, tomatoes, asparagus, spinach, to name a few. Add some grated cheese, if desired.

Canadian Bacon and Portabella Mushrooms
Use a bit of olive oil to cook diced bacon and sliced portabella. Add salt and pepper, cook until mushrooms are soft and bacon is cooked through. If you use

dairy, try splashing on a bit of cream or half-and-half and a sprinkle of Parmesan cheese (not the kind out of a green can!).

Garlic Cauliflower

Dice some steamed cauliflower and sauté in butter or olive oil along with some minced garlic, salt, pepper, and dill. If desired, add grated cheese or soy cheese.

Use your imagination to create sweet or savory crepes. Just about anything goes! Try leftover meat or fish, use dressings and sauces.

2 Crepes = 83 kcal; 8g protein; 18g carbohydrate; 4.9g fat (1g saturated) With Blintz filling: 153 kcal; 14g protein; 3g carbohydrate; 7.9g fat (2g saturated)

BASIC REAL OATMEAL

Serves 2

Cooked whole oats are an entirely different experience than quick-cooking or instant oatmeal. While whole oats take longer to cook than the refined substitutes, there are easy ways to make it equally convenient for your busy mornings.

⅔ cup **Whole Rolled Oats**
1⅓-2 cups **Water** (depending on how thick a porridge you like)
Pinch of **Salt**

Method One:
1. Place everything in the top of a double boiler. Cover.

2. Set over boiling water and allow to cook while you go about your early morning activities. Oats will be ready in about 30 minutes but can sit longer if you're not ready.

Note: Make sure you have enough water in the lower pot so it doesn't all evaporate while you're out of the kitchen. (3-4 inches should do it)

Method Two:
1. The night before, combine oats, water, and pinch of salt in a saucepan. As soon as oats come to a boil, turn off heat, cover, and let sit on stove overnight. If it's too warm to leave oats out overnight, either prepare in early evening then refrigerate or, after oats have come to a boil, transfer to a wide-mouth thermos bottle, seal, and let sit overnight.

2. In the morning, add a small amount of water or milk to prevent sticking and reheat.

> Instead of brown sugar, try sweetening the oats with stevia or Trutina®
> (see glossary), then add a few drops of maple flavoring. You can also add
> a small amount of raisins, depending on your level of tolerance for
> carbohydrates (try 1 tablespoon). If you cook the raisins with the oats,
> they will also sweeten the oatmeal.

1 serving = 104 kcal; 4g protein; 18g carbohydrate (2g fiber); 1.7g unsaturated fat

CRUSTLESS QUICHE

Serves 8

This quiche can be made ahead for a brunch or a daily breakfast. It reheats and freezes well; try freezing single pieces in plastic baggies and thawing as you need. It's a very forgiving recipe and lends itself to changes, so be creative!

8 whole **Eggs**
8 **Egg Whites***
1 tablespoon fresh **Thyme** or 1 teaspoon dried
1½ teaspoons ground **Black Pepper**
4 ounces **Neufchatel Cheese**
1 cup minced **Green Onions**
2 10-ounce packages **Frozen Spinach**, thawed and squeezed dry
    (important or quiche will be watery)
1 cup diced **Sweet Red Bell Pepper**
4 ounces low-fat **Cheddar**, grated
4 ounces low-fat **Monterey Jack**, grated

1. Blend whole eggs, egg whites, spices, and Neufchatel in blender until thoroughly mixed.

2. In large mixing bowl, combine egg mixture with all other ingredients.

3. Lightly wipe the inside of a 9" x 13" rectangular baking pan with olive oil. Pour quiche mixture in pan. Bake at 350° for 50 minutes, until a knife inserted in center comes out clean.

4. Cool, then slice into desired number of pieces. When cooled, wrap pieces in plastic wrap or place in baggies. Freeze what you won't use in 2-3 days.

1 serving = 212 kcal; 20g protein; 6g carbohydrate (2g fiber); 12.8g fat (6g saturated)

---

* For egg whites I use a product called Just Whites®, a powdered egg white with no additives. Although you do have to mix it, I find it easy to use and preferable to wasting yolks—and a lot cheaper too. Many people use a commercial egg substitute in this recipe as well. I make my own egg substitute by adding ⅛ teaspoon Xanthan Gum (available in health food stores) and ½ teaspoon turmeric for color to the whites in this recipe, but the recipe works without these additions too.

WHEY BETTER PANCAKES

Makes 12 (3-inch) pancakes

This is a rich and tasty flourless pancake that makes a nice weekend breakfast treat. Most of the fat in this recipe is healthy, unsaturated fat. Leftovers, if there are any, make a quick, easy, high-protein snack.

½ cup **Vanilla Whey Protein Powder**
2 **Eggs**
2 tablespoons **Half-and-Half** (milk can be substituted)
½ cup **Part Skim Ricotta Cheese**
2 teaspoons **Baking Powder** (aluminum-free)

1. Place all ingredients in a blender and blend until smooth and well combined.

2. Heat a skillet and lightly spray with cooking oil. Turn heat to medium low. Using a ¼ cup measure filled about ¾ full, pour 3 pancakes onto pan at a time. When cakes start to get open holes on the top side, gently flip over. These cakes cook quickly and darken easily, so don't leave them unattended.

1 pancake = 65 kcal; 9g protein; 1g carbohydrate; 1.8g fat

BLUEBERRY SAUCE
Serves 2

This is very easy to put together as pancakes are cooking and makes a flavorful alternative to maple syrup.

1 cup frozen **Blueberries**
⅛ cup **Water**
1 tablespoon **Water**
1 teaspoon **Arrowroot**
Stevia Liquid to taste

1. Place blueberries in small saucepan with ⅛ cup water over low heat until blueberries are soft and release liquid.

2. In a small bowl or cup, dissolve arrowroot in the tablespoon of water. Stir to keep arrowroot mixed. Allow berries to come to a gentle boil while stirring in arrowroot mixture. As sauce thickens, turn heat to low and allow to cook for a minute or two.

3. Sweeten with stevia to taste, starting with 3 or 4 drops.

1 serving = 56 kcal; 13g carbohydrate (2g fiber); 0.5g unsaturated fat

Variations: Use any frozen berry to make a fruit sauce—strawberries, raspberries, mixed berries—following the formula above. If you prefer a smooth raspberry, put the cooked berry mixture through a fine strainer before thickening with the arrowroot.

SPROUTED FRENCH TOAST WITH ALMOND NUT BUTTER DELIGHT

For each serving:
2 slices **Sprouted Grain Bread***
1 **Egg**
½ teaspoon **Olive Oil**
1½ tablespoons **Almond Nut Butter Delight** (page 360)
2 teaspoons **Water**
Pinch of **salt**
½ teaspoon **Cinnamon** (optional)

1. Crack open egg into shallow bowl or pan large enough to hold bread slices. Add water, salt, and cinnamon; beat egg until well-blended.

2. Heat a cast iron skillet or other frying pan on medium heat. While pan heats, soak bread in egg mixture, turning once and making sure all surfaces are coated with egg.

3. Place bread in frying pan and fry on both sides until egg is cooked and bread is firm.

4. Serve each slice with nut butter spread.

1 serving = 349 kcal; 23g protein; 38g carbohydrate (6g fiber); 11.3g fat (2g saturated)

---

*Sprouted grain bread is made from grains such as wheat berries, millet, or barley, which have been soaked and then sprouted. The sprouts are then ground, formed, and baked into bread, which although flourless, makes a delicious bread that is high in protein and low in high glycemic carbohydrates. Sprouting makes the grains more digestible, as well as vital and nutritious. Sprouted grain bread can be found in health food stores, often in a freezer case. Some brands that are called sprouted grain actually do contain milled flour as well, so read labels carefully for ingredients and carbohydrate content to find one that works for you. My favorite brand is Ezekiel Seven-Grain®.

COTTAGE CHEESE PANCAKES
Serves 2

These pancakes make a delightful weekend breakfast and are much lighter than the traditional flour-based pancake.

1 cup low-fat **Cottage Cheese**
2 **Eggs**, separated
1½ tablespoons **Arrowroot**
2 drops **Stevia Liquid**
½ teaspoon **Vanilla Extract** (or try Lemon, Orange extracts)
¼ teaspoon **Salt**
½ teaspoon **Cinnamon** (optional)
Olive Oil for cooking

1. Stir together all ingredients except egg whites.

2. Beat egg whites until they form stiff peaks. Fold into the cottage cheese mixture gently to incorporate without breaking down the whites.

3. Heat a skillet (cast iron works well) and when hot, add just enough oil to coat bottom. Drop batter by tablespoons. Cook on one side until puffed up and pancake holds together when you slip a spatula underneath. Flip over and cook on other side until lightly browned.

Serve with blueberry or fruit sauce (page 257) or unsweetened applesauce.

1 serving = 202 kcal; 21g protein; 10g carbohydrate; 7.2g fat (2g saturated)
Nutritional information for topping is on page 257.

SALAD DRESSINGS, SAUCES, AND MARINADES

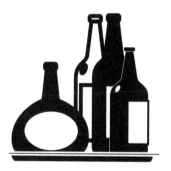

ESSENTIAL HERB VINAIGRETTE

Makes 1¾ cups

This dressing is an easy way to get some Omega 3 fat in your diet every day. It can easily be used for salads or vegetables, or to marinate chicken, beef, or fish. Getting fat into your diet in a raw, unheated form is the most healthful way to give your body the fat it needs to function optimally.

½ cup **Extra Virgin Olive Oil**
½ cup **Flaxseed Oil**
¾ cup **Cider or Balsamic Vinegar**
1 tablespoon **Dijon or Stoneground Mustard**
1-2 large clove(s) **Garlic**, crushed
½ teaspoon **Lemon Pepper** (use regular pepper if not available)
1 teaspoon **Basil**
1 teaspoon **Parsley**
½ teaspoon **Marjoram**
½ teaspoon **Thyme**
Salt to taste
1-2 drops **Stevia Liquid (optional)**

Mix all ingredients in a blender. Store in glass jar in refrigerator.

1 tablespoon = 67 kcal; 8.1g unsaturated fat

Note: The stevia is used to cut the sharpness of the dressing, which some people don't like. Omit if you like.

GREEK SALAD DRESSING
Makes 1 cup

5 tablespoons **Olive Oil**
¼ cup **Water**
2 tablespoons **White Wine Vinegar**
1 tablespoon **Oregano**
2 tablespoons fresh **Lemon Juice**
½ teaspoon **Sea Salt**
½ teaspoon **Black Pepper**
2 cloves **Garlic**, crushed

1.   Combine all ingredients in jar.

2.   Shake well. Make ahead of time to allow flavors to develop.

1 tablespoon = 54 kcal; 6g unsaturated fat

SIMPLE VINAIGRETTE (REDUCED FAT)
Makes 1¼ cups

½ cup **Olive Oil** (or ¼ cup each flaxseed and olive oils)
1 cup **Balsamic Vinegar or Red Wine Vinegar**
1 clove **Garlic**, crushed
½ teaspoon **Basil**
½ teaspoon **Oregano**
¼ teaspoon **Thyme**

Mix ingredients together in a pint jar and store in refrigerator. Use for salads, steamed vegetables, or as a marinade.

1 tablespoon = 68 kcal; 6.8g unsaturated fat

I'm not an advocate of low-fat diets; I think people need moderate amounts of healthful fat in their diet for optimal health, unless there is some reason their bodies are unable to metabolize fat. But in a meal or a day that other-wise contains adequate fat sources, a lower-fat dressing can come in handy.

LEMON MISO TAHINI DRESSING
Makes 2 cups

This dressing makes a creamy topping for salads, steamed vegetables, or an occasional baked potato. Sesame seeds in the tahini are a good source of calcium as well as providing a healthful source of fat to the diet.

½ cup **Tahini**
1 cup **Filtered Water,** boiling
1 tablespoon **Light Miso***
3 tablespoons fresh **Lemon Juice**
2 tablespoons chopped **Scallions**
2 cloves **Garlic,** crushed
1 teaspoon **Dill Weed**

Blend all ingredients together. Store in glass jar in refrigerator. Use on salads or as a topping/dip for steamed or raw veggies. Will keep for about 2 weeks.

1 tablespoon = 26 kcal; 1g carbohydrate; 2.1g unsaturated fat

---

*Miso is a fermented soybean paste that is used for soups in Japanese restaurants, but is also a delicious and healthful addition to dressings, marinades, and sauces. Look for it in a refrigerated case in your health food grocery store.

MUSTARD APPLE VINAIGRETTE

Makes 1 cup

A sweet, tangy dressing for those who like a mustard–honey type of dressing but don't want all the sugar.

¼ cup **Olive Oil**
¼ cup **Cider Vinegar**
2 tablespoons **Dijon Mustard**
½ small, peeled **Apple**, sweet variety, seeds and core removed, chopped
¼ cup **Water**
Stevia Liquid (optional)

1. Place oil and vinegar in blender and blend on high until combined. Add apple pieces and mustard, blend until completely smooth. Add water.

2. If you like a sweeter dressing, add 2-3 drops of stevia liquid or to taste.

1 tablespoon = 34 kcal; 0.5g carbohydrate; 3.4g unsaturated fat

UME ALMOND DIP OR DRESSING
Makes 1½ cups

This is an unusual dip that's a hit at parties, served with lightly steamed vegetables. It has a tangy, rich flavor that contrasts well with lightly cooked vegetables. The recipe comes from Meredith McCarty's Fresh From the Vegetarian Kitchen. It may seem strange at first glance, but I encourage you to give it a try!

2 tablespoons **Umeboshi Plum Paste***
4 tablespoons **Almond Butter**
½ medium **Onion**, coarsely chopped
1 cup **Water**

1. Place all ingredients except water in blender or food processor and blend, stopping occasionally to scrape down sides.

2. Add water slowly until desired consistency is reached (will thicken a lot as it chills). Store in refrigerator. Will keep 7-10 days.

¼ **cup** = 52 kcal; 2g carbohydrate; 4.4g unsaturated fat

---

*Umeboshi plums are a salty Japanese plum believed in Oriental medicine to have great medicinal properties; they also add an unusual but delicious taste to food. The plums can be purchased whole or as a paste. Because they are very salty, only a small amount is used at one time. Once opened, both plums and paste should be stored in refrigerator. Find these in a health food store in the macrobiotic section.

NUTRITION MAGICIAN'S BARBECUE SAUCE

Makes 1 cup

At last, a barbecue sauce without sugar or refined sweeteners that has a rich taste and tang with a tiny bit of heat! I usually double or quadruple the recipe—it keeps forever in the refrigerator and you can use it for meatballs, chicken, tempeh, ground beef, or anyplace else you want the flavor of barbecue.

¼ cup **Cider Vinegar**

¼ cup **Tamari**

¼ cup **Tomato Paste**

1 tablespoon **Olive Oil**

2 tablespoons **Raisins**

¼ cup **Water**

1 tablespoon **Dry Mustard**

½ tablespoon **Black Pepper**

⅛ - ¼ teaspoon **Red Pepper Flakes**

2 large cloves **Garlic,** crushed

½ teaspoon **Maple Extract**

15 drops **Stevia Liquid**

2-3 drops **Liquid (Hickory or Mesquite) Smoke**

1. Place raisins and water in small saucepan, bring to a boil, then simmer covered, several minutes. Remove from heat and allow to sit covered.

2. Assemble remaining ingredients in blender, then add softened raisins and liquid. Blend until completely smooth. Store in glass jar in refrigerator. Keeps for a long time.

¼ **cup** = 70 kcal; 2g protein; 9g carbohydrate (1g fiber); 3.6g unsaturated fat

ASIAN MARINADE

Makes ¾ cup

For chicken, fish, tempeh, etc.

¼ cup **Cider Vinegar**
2 tablespoons **Toasted Sesame Oil**
2 tablespoons **Tamari or Soy Sauce**
¼ cup **Orange Juice**
1 tablespoon **Orange Juice Concentrate**
1-inch piece **Ginger Root,** coarsely chopped (peeling not necessary)
2 medium to large **Garlic Cloves,** minced or pressed
6 drops **Stevia Liquid** (adjust to taste)

Combine all ingredients in a blender or food processor until well mixed.

2 tablespoons = 57 kcal; 3g carbohydrate; 4.6g unsaturated fat

SOUTHEAST ASIAN PINEAPPLE SESAME DRESSING

Makes ¾ cup

From Moosewood Restaurant Low-Fat Favorites, *this makes a particularly good flavorful and slightly sweet marinade for vegetables, or it can be used to dress up fish, chicken, or tempeh.*

¼ cup **Unsweetened Crushed Pineapple**
1 tablespoon **Light Miso** (such as barley, chickpea, shiro)
1 tablespoon **Tamari or Soy Sauce**
1 tablespoon **Rice Vinegar**
1 tablespoon **Sesame Oil**
1 clove **Garlic**
¼ cup **Water or Unsweetened Pineapple Juice**

Place all ingredients in blender or food processor and purée until smooth.

3 tablespoons = 59 kcal; 1g protein; 5g carbohydrate; 3.7g unsaturated fat

JAMAICAN JERK SAUCE

Makes 1 cup

This Caribbean-influenced sauce is great with pork, chicken, fish, tofu, or tempeh. Adapted from a recipe in The Moosewood Restaurant Low-fat Favorites, *I replaced the original recipe's sugar with stevia to trim the carbohydrates while retaining the needed sweetness.*

1 small to medium **Onion**, coarsely chopped (about ½ cup)
3 fresh **Green Chilies** (about 8 or 9 inches altogether)
3 tablespoons **Tamari or Soy Sauce**
¼ cup **Balsamic Vinegar**
8-12 drops **Stevia Liquid** (adjust to taste)
2 teaspoons fresh grated **Ginger Root**
2 cloves **Garlic**, minced or pressed
1 teaspoon **Thyme**
1 teaspoon **Cloves**
1 teaspoon **Cinnamon**
½ teaspoon **Black Pepper**

1. Place all ingredients in a blender starting with 8 drops of stevia. Blend until smooth.

2. Adjust stevia to taste if needed. Store in glass jar in refrigerator.

¼ **cup** = 49 kcal; 2g protein; 9g carbohydrate (1g fiber); 0.3g unsaturated fat

---

For a sauce with mild heat that "nips" but doesn't bite, split the chilies and remove the pith (soft membrane) and seeds. Be sure to wear rubber gloves when cutting and handling chilies. Combine all ingredients except stevia in a blender and mix until a smooth purée. Add stevia to taste.

SOUPS

LOW-CARB PORTUGUESE KALE AND SAUSAGE SOUP

Serves 4

Even without the traditional potatoes this is still a great fall and winter soup, and it's a snap to make. This recipe makes a hearty meal in a bowl.

1¾ pounds **Italian Turkey Sausage** removed from casing (use hot or sweet or a combination)
1 pound **Kale,** stripped from stems
1 cup chopped **Onion**
1 cup **Carrots** in matchsticks*
2 cloves **Garlic,** minced or crushed
1 tablespoon **Olive Oil**
4 cups **Chicken Stock**
6 tablespoons grated **Parmesan Cheese**, optional

1. Put oil in heated, heavy soup pot. Sauté onions and garlic for several minutes.

2. Chop kale into small pieces and place in boiling water; simmer for 4 minutes, then drain.

3. Add turkey sausage to onions and garlic. Break up pieces with spoon while stirring. When sausage is browned, add carrot sticks and sauté all for 10 more minutes.

4. Add stock, heat to boil, then reduce heat to simmer until carrots are barely tender. Remove from heat; add cooked kale, and let sit 10 minutes before serving. Season to taste with salt and pepper.

Serve with 1-2 tablespoons grated Parmesan per serving, if desired

2 cups = 413 kcal; 34g protein; 21g carbohydrate (4g fiber); 20.7g fat (4g saturated)
2 cups (w/parmesan) = 444 kcal; 37g protein; 21g carbohydrate (4g fiber); 22.9g fat (6g saturated)

*Cut carrots into matchsticks by first slicing them on the diagonal into ¾-inch slices. Spread the slices apart slightly and cut into ¼-inch sticks.

CREAM OF ANY VEGETABLE SOUP

Serves 6

A small amount of rolled oats and a blender give these soups their creamy texture without the traditional milk, cream, or flour used to make cream soup. The result is a rich-tasting but light soup that can be varied endlessly.

½ to 1 cup chopped **Onions**
4 cups chopped **Asparagus Stems**
1 cup **AsparagusTips**, steamed 3-4 minutes
⅓ cup **Rolled Oats**
1 tablespoon **Sesame Oil**
3-5 cups **Stock or Water**
½ teaspoon **Nutmeg**
Salt and Pepper to taste

1. Heat a heavy-bottomed soup pot; when hot, add sesame oil then chopped onions. Sauté and stir 3-5 minutes.

2. Add asparagus stems and pinch of salt. Stir and cook another few minutes.

3. Add oats and 3 cups stock or water. Bring to a boil, cover, reduce heat, and simmer 15 minutes.

4. Purée mixture in blender until smooth. Return to pot and add stock until soup is desired consistency. Bring to boil again then reduce heat to simmer.

5. Add nutmeg and adjust salt and pepper to taste. Add asparagus tips; simmer just until tips turn bright green, then serve.

1 serving (approximately 1 cup) = 88 kcal; 4g protein; 12g carbohydrate (4g fiber); 3g unsaturated fat

---

Variations:
Cream of Broccoli: Follow key recipe using ½ cup onion, ½ cup celery, 1-2 cloves garlic, and 4 cups chopped broccoli in place of asparagus. Garnish each bowl with a few lightly steamed broccoli florets and a sprinkling of grated Parmesan or Swiss cheese.

Cream of Carrot: Follow key recipe using ½ cup onion, ½ cup celery, 4 cups carrots. Substitute 1 teaspoon thyme or tarragon for nutmeg. Garnish with thinly sliced scallions. Lightly steamed carrot flowers also make a nice garnish.

Cream of Mushroom: Clean and trim 1 pound of fresh mushrooms. Chop the stems and dice the caps. Sauté stems with onions. Add 3 cups stock or water, pinch of salt, and ⅓ cup oatmeal and cook 15 minutes. Purée and return to pot. Add diced caps, 1-2 bay leaves, substitute a teaspoon thyme or tarragon for nutmeg, and simmer 10 minutes. Remove bay leaves. Garnish with chopped parsley or thinly sliced scallions.

Cream of Cauliflower: Follow key recipe using olive oil instead of sesame oil. Use leeks and a clove of garlic in place of onion and 4 cups cauliflower in place of asparagus. Use olive oil in place of sesame oil, and 1 teaspoon dried dill in place of nutmeg. Use minimum amount of stock to keep consistency thicker.

CURRIED CREAM OF CAULIFLOWER SOUP

Serves 4

When I am eating this soup, I love it more than anything in the world! This is a very rich soup, so a smaller serving than you might usually have is quite satisfying.

2 teaspoons **Butter**
½ cup chopped **Onion**
1 tablespoon **Curry Powder** (This amount gives a little bite; use less if you prefer)
⅛ teaspoon **Saffron**
½ cup **Golden Delicious** or other sweet apple, seeded and chopped
3 cups **Cauliflower florets**
2 cups **Vegetable or Chicken Broth**, warmed
½ cup **Lite Coconut Milk**

1.   Melt butter in heavy pot over medium heat. Sauté onions, curry, and saffron for 2 minutes stirring often.

2.   Add apple and sauté another 5 minutes.

3.   Add cauliflower, warm stock, salt, and pepper to taste. Bring to boil, then reduce to simmer and cook until cauliflower is tender, 15-20 minutes.

4.   Add coconut milk and simmer until hot. Transfer in batches to a blender and purée until smooth.

¾ **cup** = 73 kcal; 2g protein; 9g carbohydrate (3g fiber); 4g fat (2g saturated)

CREAMY ZUCCHINI SOUP

Serves 8

This recipe is originally from Lorna Sass' Cooking Under Pressure, a great pressure cooker cookbook. It's been adapted here for stovetop preparation, and I've cut back the fat slightly. It's a wonderful comfort food—warm, creamy, and flavorful.

1 tablespoon **Olive Oil**
1 large **Onion**, coarsely chopped (about 1½ cups)
2 large **Garlic Cloves**, crushed
2 small **Potatoes** (totaling ½ pound), scrubbed and cut into ½-inch dice
2 large **Carrots,** cut in ½-inch slices
4 cups **Vegetable Stock**
6 medium **Zucchini** (2 pounds), cut in 1-inch chunks
1 tablespoon fresh **Basil** or 1 teaspoon dried
Salt and freshly ground **Pepper** to taste

1. Cut up all the vegetables.

2. Heat a large soup pot; when heated, add the olive oil. Sauté onion and garlic while stirring for one minute. Add the potato and sauté 1-2 minutes more. If vegetables stick, add a few tablespoons of the stock.

3. Add remaining ingredients and stir to blend. Cover, bring to boil, reduce heat, and simmer until all the vegetables are easily pierced with fork, about 12-15 minutes. Allow soup to cool slightly.

4. Use blender or food processor to purée soup in batches. Season to taste with salt and pepper.

1 cup = 75 kcal; 2g protein; 13g carbohydrate (3g fiber); 1.9g unsaturated fat

MORNING SOUP

Serves 2

This soup is easy to assemble and fresh. I like it on cold mornings when I want something filling and warming, but light. It's actually great for any meal, but I made it up one morning when I wanted a meal that would fuel me for a couple hours' work before I went to work out, hence the name. If you're not sure about the idea of vegetables for breakfast, try this tasty recipe!

3 cups **Chicken Stock**
4 **Eggs**, whisked in a small bowl
2 cups **Shredded Cabbage** (can use prepackaged for convenience)
2 handfuls fresh **Mung Bean Sprouts**
4 tablespoons **Chopped Scallions**
Salt and Pepper to taste
3 tablespoons grated **Parmesan Cheese** (optional)

1. Bring chicken stock to a boil. Add cabbage and reduce heat to a simmer. Simmer covered for 10 minutes until cabbage is soft.

2. Add mung bean sprouts and scallions, and then drizzle beaten egg over soup. Cook until egg is set, about 1 minute. Stir in Parmesan cheese. Serve immediately.

1 serving = 281 kcal; 25g protein; 10g carbohydrate (2g fiber); 14.3g fat (5g saturated)

CREAMY LEEK AND FAUXTATO SOUP

Serves 6

My sister, who inspires much of what I do, came up with this low-carbohydrate remake of an old, cold-weather standard. The pinch of cayenne is optional but gives the soup a nice, warming undertone without making it spicy.

2 tablespoons **Butter**
6 medium **Leeks**, white part only, well rinsed*
3 stalks **Celery**, sliced thinly
4 cups **Cauliflower** florets (about a 6-inch diameter head of cauliflower, trimmed)
5 cups **Chicken or Vegetable Stock**
¼ cup finely minced fresh **Dill**
Salt and Pepper to taste
Pinch of **Cayenne** (optional)

1. Melt butter in heavy-bottomed soup pot. Sauté leeks for 5 minutes, stirring occasionally. Add celery and cook 3 minutes more.

2. Add cauliflower and stock. Bring to a boil, reduce heat, cover and simmer about 20 minutes until cauliflower is soft when pierced with a fork.

3. Cool slightly. Purée solids with some liquid in batches in blender until consistency is smooth. Place blended batches in storage container; add stock just until desired consistency is reached. (Save any remaining stock for another use.) Add dill, salt and pepper, and cayenne.

> *To thoroughly wash leeks, first trim off the root end. Make a vertical slit in the white part of the leek that goes about ⅔ of the way through the root. Gently pull the root open while running under cool water to remove any dirt particles that may be trapped inside.

1 serving = 165 kcal; 7g protein; 22g carbohydrate (4g fiber); 5.6g fat (2g saturated)

GARDEN GASPACHO

Serves 6

Good gaspacho in the summer is a heavenly way to eat your vegetables!

1½ slices **Sprouted Grain Bread,** torn into crumbs
3 tablespoons **Red Wine Vinegar**
2 cloves **Garlic,** crushed
2 tablespoons **Olive Oil**
1 large **Cucumber**, seeded and chopped
1 **Green Bell Pepper**, chopped into small pieces
1 ripe **Avocado**, cut into small pieces
8 large, ripe **Tomatoes**, peeled, seeded, and chopped*
1 cup cold **Water**
¼ cup fresh **Basil**
Salt and Pepper to taste

1. In a medium-sized mixing bowl, mash the breadcrumbs with the oil, vinegar, and garlic to make a smooth paste. Set aside.

2. Seed the cucumber by peeling and slicing in half lengthwise. Use a teaspoon to scrape out the seeds from each half. Cut into small pieces and set aside. To cut the avocado, slice in half all the way around and remove pit. Score the meat on each half, vertically and horizontally, then use a spoon to gently remove pieces into the bowl with the cucumbers.

3. Blend the tomatoes in a blender or food processor until only small chunks remain.

4. Mix the tomatoes and all other vegetables together. Add ½ cup to the paste and blend until well mixed, then add remaining tomato and vegetable mixture and the cold water. Add basil, salt, and pepper to taste. Tastes best if allowed to sit in refrigerator overnight.

1 serving = 122 kcal; 1g protein; 8g carbohydrate (3g fiber); 9.8g fat (1g saturated)

> *To peel fresh tomatoes, drop into boiling water for a minute or two until skins begin to crack. Remove, run under cold water, and slip skins off. Or, for a quicker gaspacho, use one 28-ounce can of whole or diced tomatoes, including juice.

> **Spanish Meatballs:** Season a pound of lean ground beef with salt, pepper, and 2 teaspoons of chili powder (more or less to taste). Form about 18 small meatballs, place in 2 cups of gaspacho in a wide pot. Bring to a boil then turn heat down to a simmer. Simmer meatballs for 20 minutes.

SALADS

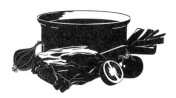

GIMME FIVE CHEF'S SALAD

Serves 2

Eating a big salad for lunch is one way to easily get in at least five servings of nutrient- and phytochemical-rich vegetables. More importantly, though, is that with a tiny bit of preparation, salads are a satisfying, easy-to-make meal that can always be varied.

3 cups **Romaine Lettuce**
3 cups **Baby Spinach Leaves or Mixed Greens**
½ large **Carrot**, grated
1 cup **Grape or Cherry Tomatoes**
1 **Red or Green Bell Pepper** (or half of each), seeded and chopped
1 **Cucumber**, sliced (peeled if waxed)
2 6-ounce cans of **Tuna**, drained, **or** 9 ounces deli **Turkey** or **Ham**, **or** 2 ounces **Cheese** and 6 ounces **Turkey** or **Ham**
1½ tablespoons **Raisins** (optional)
1½ tablespoons **Sunflower or Pumpkin Seeds*** (optional)

1 serving with 4 ounces tuna = 265 kcal; 20g protein; 26g carbohydrate (8g fiber); 5.3g unsaturated fat

---

*Try toasting the seeds first in a dry frying pan over medium heat for several minutes until they begin to brown and give off a fragrant smell. Shake or stir periodically while toasting so they don't burn. Toast extra (enough for a week or two) and keep in a sealed jar.

FENNEL, APPLE, AND WALNUT SALAD WITH BLUE CHEESE
Serves 2

3 cups **Romaine Lettuce**, torn into bite-sized pieces
1 cup **Diced Fennel** (use bulb and stalk)
2 tablespoons **Toasted Walnuts**, chopped*
2 ounces **Blue Cheese,** crumbled
1 medium **Apple**, (crisp, tart variety such as Braeburn, Granny Smith, Winesap)

1. Core and dice the apple into ½-inch pieces.

2. Combine all ingredients. Serve with an olive oil
   and vinegar dressing such as Essential Herb Vinaigrette.

1 serving = 213 kcal; 9g protein; 19g carbohydrate (3g fiber); 12.4g fat (5g saturated)

---

*Toast walnuts or any nut by stirring for several minutes in a dry frying pan over medium heat. Nuts will begin to smell fragrant when done. Store in a glass jar.

THAI MUNG BEAN SALAD

Serves 8

This is a crunchy salad with a bit of zip to it. It makes a nice side to fish or chicken dishes that have ginger, tamari, or sesame oil as seasonings.

1 pound fresh **Mung Bean Sprouts**, rinsed and drained well
1 cup **Carrots**, raw or parboiled, cut into matchstick pieces (see box on page 272)
1 **Cucumber**, peeled if waxed or not organic
½ cup minced, fresh **Cilantro**
2 tablespoons toasted and chopped **Peanuts** (see box on page 281)

Dressing:
⅓ cup **Rice Vinegar** (no sugar added)
1 tablespoon **Tamari**
2 tablespoons **Toasted Sesame Oil**
2 tablespoons **Walnut Oil**
3 drops **Stevia Liquid**
½ teaspoon dried **Red Chili Pepper Flakes**

1. In large salad bowl, place the mung sprouts and the carrots. Prepare the cucumber by running the tines of a fork down the length of it, all around, to create indented lines. Slice the cucumber into thin slices. Toss all the vegetables together.

2. Blend the dressing ingredients together; just before serving, toss dressing with the vegetables.

3. Garnish salad with fresh cilantro and chopped peanuts.

1 serving = 95 kcal; 2g protein; 6g carbohydrate (1g fiber); 7.4g unsaturated fat

JICAMA ORANGE SALAD

Serves 4

Jicama is a large tuber with a tough, dull-brown skin. Peel the skin and find a sweet and crunchy treat. This is an unusual and very refreshing salad.

12 ounces (¾ pound) **Jicama**, peeled and cut into matchsticks
2 **Navel Oranges**, peeled, white membrane removed
12 **Black Pitted Olives**, sliced into rings
½ cup sliced **Red Onion**
2 tablespoons **Olive Oil**
1½ tablespoons fresh **Lemon Juice**
¼ teaspoon **Cumin**

1. Toss onion, jicama, and olives in medium-sized bowl. In small bowl blend oil, lemon juice, and cumin until combined. Pour over vegetables and toss again to coat.

2. Cut oranges in half lengthwise. Slice halves into ¼-inch semi-circles. Combine with jicama and mix gently to combine.

1 serving = 88 kcal; 1g protein; 10g carbohydrate (1g fiber); 5.4g unsaturated fat

BACON, LETTUCE, AND TOMATO SALAD

Serves 2

When I reduced my refined carbohydrate consumption, I missed having BLT's. I find this salad gives me all the great tastes without the ill effects I'd get from the bread.

4 cups **Romaine or other Lettuce**
½ cup **Cherry Tomatoes** cut in half
4 slices **Cooked Bacon or Turkey Bacon** (cured without sugar)
4 ounces **Smoked Mozzarella**, cut in small cubes

1. Rinse and tear lettuce and divide on two plates.

2. Top with sliced tomatoes, crumbled bacon, and cheese. Use dressing of choice.

1 serving (not including dressing) =
with Turkey Bacon: 246 kcal; 21g protein; 7g carbohydrate (3 fiber); 10.2g fat (5g saturated)
with Pork Bacon: 250 kcal; 20g protein; 8g carbohydrate (3g fiber); 14.2g fat (7g saturated)

FIRECRACKER SLAW

Serves 4

My friend Scott Mann made up this great variation on coleslaw for a party and allowed me the honor of naming it!

3 cups thinly shredded **Purple Cabbage**
1 **Sweet Red Bell Pepper**, thinly sliced
1 small **Carrot**, finely diced
1-2 teaspoons minced **Hot Finger Peppers** (use gloves to handle)
1½ tablespoons **Dried Currants**
1½ tablespoons **Olive Oil**
Juice of 1 **Lime**
½ cup finely chopped, fresh **Cilantro**
Salt and Pepper to taste

1. Toss together the vegetables, currants, and hot pepper.

2. Add salt and pepper, olive oil, and lime juice. Mix well.

3. Allow to sit an hour or so before serving. Toss with ½ cup fresh chopped cilantro before serving.

1 cup = 77 kcal; 1g protein; 7.5g carbohydrate (1g fiber); 5.3g unsaturated fat

MARINATED VEGETABLE SALAD

Serves 4

Even though this is a great way to use odd bits of vegetables, don't think of this only as a leftover salad. When you have steamed or par-boiled vegetables in your refrigerator, marinating a combination of them is a quick and easy way to have a lunch or snack item on hand.

1. From the lists below, combine **6 cups of vegetables.**

2. Gently toss together in bowl with ⅓ cup of **Essential Herb Vinaigrette** (page 262).

3. If desired, add 1 cup **sliced black and green olives.**

4. Store in container with tight-fitting lid that will allow you to turn vegetables over periodically to thoroughly marinate all the vegetables.

Parboiled Vegetables

Drop vegetables, one kind at a time, into boiling water for 1 minute. Then plunge into ice water to stop cooking. Cook vegetables in order from the weakest flavored ones to the strongest. Vegetables should retain bright color and crispness.

Zucchini rounds or sticks
Summer Squash rounds or sticks
Green or Yellow String Beans
Brussel Sprouts (need longer cooking)
Broccoli crowns and peeled stems in rounds or sticks

Cauliflower
Asparagus
Cabbage chunks

Tip: Use a vegetable peeler to remove tough outer skin of broccoli stems. Once peeled, the stems are a good addition to any vegetable dish, soup, or stir-fry.

Raw Vegetables
Daikon Radish slices
Jicama, peeled and cut into sticks
Green Bell Peppers, seeded and chopped
Grape or Cherry Tomatoes
Red, Yellow, Orange Bell Peppers, seeded and chopped
Cucumbers, peeled, seeded, and sliced (seeding will help them keep better)

Celery, sliced diagonally
Mushrooms, cut in half
Red Radish slices
Carrot rounds

Nutritional count will depend on specific combination, but typically, 1½ cups of low-glycemic vegetables will provide about 15g carbohydrate, of which 4 or 5 will be fiber grams.

MATABANIC GREEK SALAD WITH ROASTED RED BEETS

Serves 2

Twice a year for the last 12 years I've gone on a work/play retreat with the same group of colleagues. We all share in food preparation for the weekends. This variation on traditional Greek Salad, one of my contributions, is one of our favorite lunches. The roasted red beets were a recent adaptation by one of our group. Most people have never had bok choy, a type of chinese cabbage, but uncooked it makes a refreshing, crunchy addition to any salad.

4-6 cups **Romaine Lettuce**, torn into bite-sized pieces
2 cups sliced **Bok Choy**, stalk and leaves
½ **Green Bell Pepper**, seeded and sliced
½ **Red Bell Pepper**, seeded and sliced
3 **Pickling Cucumbers**, sliced
1 cup **Grape Tomatoes**
Thinly sliced **Red Onion** to taste
12-14 **Kalamata Olives**
3 ounces **Feta Cheese**
1 cup **Roasted Red Beets***, cut into wedges

1.	Combine and toss all ingredients except beets and feta cheese.

2.	Arrange beets on top of each portion and sprinkle with crumbled feta cheese.

1 serving = 133 kcals; 6g protein; 14g carbohydrate (4g fiber); 6.6g fat (3.5 saturated)

---

*To roast red beets use beets that are 2½ to 3 inches diameter. Scrub but do not trim. Place in covered casserole and roast at 375° for 1½ hours or until you can pierce easily with a knife. Allow beets to cool, then remove skin. I like to slice in half lengthwise then cut into small wedges, but any shape that suits you will be fine.

ASIAN-STYLE BROCCOLI SLAW
Serves 4

1 package **Broccoli Slaw***
1 recipe **Southeast Asian Pineapple Sesame Dressing** (below)
2 ounces (4½ tablespoons) **Pumpkin Seeds**

1. In metal or nonreactive bowl, toss broccoli slaw with dressing to taste.

2. Place pumpkin seeds in dry skillet and stir over medium-low heat until fragrant. You may also toast by placing on cookie sheet in 200° oven for about 15-20 minutes, shaking pan occasionally.

3. Add seeds just before serving so they remain crisp.

> *Broccoli slaw is made from the shredded stalks of broccoli. It is often sold pre-packaged in the produce section. If not, you can easily make it by peeling the stalks of broccoli with a vegetable peeler and running them through your food processor using the shredding disk.

SOUTHEAST ASIAN PINEAPPLE SESAME DRESSING
Makes ¾ cup
From Moosewood Restaurant Low-Fat Favorites

¼ cup **Unsweetened Crushed Pineapple**
1 tablespoon **Light Miso** (such as barley, chickpea, shiro)
1 tablespoon **Tamari**
1 tablespoon **Rice Vinegar**
1 tablespoon **Sesame Oil**
1 clove **Garlic**
¼ cup **Water or Juice from Pineapple**

Place all ingredients in blender or food processor and purée until smooth.

3 tablespoons = 50 kcals; 4g carbohydrate; 3.4g unsaturated fat

VEGETABLES

BASIC KALE OR COLLARD GREENS

Serves 4

Kale and Collards are two kinds of greens that most people barely recognize, much less eat. But both are easy to prepare, very tasty, full of fiber, and a tremendous source of nutrients, most notably calcium. A cup of cooked greens provides about 25 percent of the daily calcium needs for a woman. I have also found that if I've been indulging in food with sugar, eating some of these greens daily seems to help break the craving cycle.

1 bunch **Kale or Collard Greens**
Pinch **Salt**
Water

1. Wash the leaves.

2. In a large pot, bring about 2 inches of water with a pinch of salt to a boil.

3. Using a sharp knife (a 10-inch chef's knife works well), slice the green away from the thick center rib on both sides. (The rib can either be discarded or cut into thin slices and added to the leaves for cooking.)

4. Cut up the leaves into smaller pieces of about 2-3 inches square.

5. Place the leaves in the boiling water. Stir once or twice to get leaves to settle into the water. When water returns to a boil, turn heat down to a simmer, leaving pot uncovered.

6. Cook kale for 5-8 minutes, until tender but not mushy. Collards need slightly less time, about 4-6 minutes.

1 cup Kale = 42 kcal; 2g protein; 7g carbohydrate (3g fiber); 1g unsaturated fat
1 cup Collards = 34 kcal; 2g protein; 8g carbohydrate (3g fiber)

What does it look like? Kale is dark green and sturdy looking with a very large curly leaf growing on either side of about a 10- to 12-inch-thick stem. Collard greens have a similar center, but the leaf is large, flat, and always reminds me of a southern lady's hand-held fan!

Tips for use: I love them plain, as a complement to meals that may have other distinct flavors. But they can also be dressed up with addition of a dressing such as Essential Herb Vinaigrette (page 262) or Lemon Miso Tahini (page 264). Or, look at the Sautéed Greens Medley recipe on next page.

For a different visual effect, use thin strips of collard greens to cover the bottom of the plate and serve other items on top of it. To make these, (a technique called *chiffonade*,) after you strip the leaf off its rib, roll each half leaf up, and then slice through the roll making ½-inch-wide strips. These will cook more quickly than larger pieces, so reduce your cooking time by a minute or two.

SAUTÉED GREENS MEDLEY
Serves 4

1 pound **Greens** (any combination of Kale, Collards, Mustard, Dandelion, etc.)
1 medium **Onion**, sliced in moon-shaped wedges
2 cloves **Garlic**, minced
1 teaspoon **Olive Oil**
1 teaspoon **Sesame Oil**
Tamari* and Rice Vinegar** to taste

1. Put about 2 inches water in wide pot, add pinch of salt, cover and bring to boil. While water boils, wash greens and trim kale and collards from center rib. Chop greens into bite-sized pieces.

2. Put greens in boiling water, let water return to boil, then reduce heat. Leaving cover off, cook about 6 minutes for kale and collards, 4 minutes for mustard greens.

3. Drain greens and press with back of spoon to release excess moisture.

4. Heat heavy skillet, add olive oil. Add onions and sauté 2 minutes. Add minced garlic and continue to sauté several minutes until onions soften and begin to brown.

5. Add greens and continue cooking 2-3 minutes until greens are heated through. Sprinkle with tamari and/or rice vinegar to taste.

1 serving = 109 kcal; 4g protein; 18g carbohydrate (4g fiber); 3.2g unsaturated fat

---

*Tamari is aged soy sauce that has no preservatives or flavorings (such as MSG) added to it. It can be purchased wheat-free as well (soy sauce contains wheat).

**Look for Brown Rice Vinegar in the health food store. Most commercial rice vinegar sold in Asian markets will contain sugar.

ROASTED ROOT VEGETABLES

Serves 4-6

Root vegetables are totally underutilized as far as I'm concerned. They offer so many different flavors, a cornucopia of nutrients and phytochemicals, and a natural sweetness that can round out a meal. This savory combination is a real comfort food for fall and winter.

2½ pounds **Mixed Root Vegetables** (parsnips, beets, carrots, turnips, onions, sweet potato, rutabaga)

1 **head of Garlic**, cloves separated but not peeled

4 3-inch sprigs fresh **Rosemary**

3 **Bay Leaves**

1-2 tablespoons **Olive Oil**

2 tablespoons **Tamari**

¼ teaspoon **Pepper**

1. Preheat oven to 450°. Scrub the vegetables. Peel parsnips, onions, and rutabaga. Cut into equal-sized pieces except for parsnip, sweet potato, and carrot. Make these slightly larger, as they cook faster.

2. Toss vegetables, garlic cloves, and herbs with oil and tamari to coat. Season with pepper.

3. Put everything in a casserole large enough for vegetables to spread out. Bake 20 minutes, uncovered, in top third of oven.

4. Reduce temperature to 375°. Continue baking until tender when pierced with fork, about 20-30 minutes longer. Remove bay leaves. Garlic will be roasted in skin and can easily be "popped out" before or after serving.

Nutritional count will depend on vegetable combination.

What are they?

Root vegetables are the dense, sweet vegetables that grow in the ground— they're the root of the plant, hence the name. They include beets, carrots, parsnip, rutabaga, turnip, potato, sweet potato, and yam. Radishes are also root vegetables, but are less dense, less sugary, and contain more water.

Root vegetables (except radishes) have more impact on blood sugar than above-ground vegetables, so should be used more sparingly by those needing to regulate their blood-sugar levels closely. But don't avoid them—root vegetables can help satisfy your craving for a sweet taste in a healthful way, and also have lots of nutrients and health-protective phytochemicals.

BASIC VEGETABLE STIR-FRY
Serves 2-4

There is something incredibly satisfying about a good stir-fry. People don't often make them because of the cutting and chopping involved, but if you follow the "component cooking" guidelines in Chapter Nine, you'll have almost all the work done ahead of time with precut and parboiled vegetables.

Oils: Sesame or Walnut Oil for an Asian flavor, Olive Oil for an herb flavor.

Vegetables: Your favorite assortment of vegetables cut into bite-sized pieces. Keep vegetables separate from each other, as you will add them according to how long they take to cook.

Choose 4-6 cups from: broccoli, cauliflower, carrots, onions, scallions, leeks, green (or red, yellow, or orange) peppers, celery, asparagus, snow or sugar snap peas, mushrooms, mung bean sprouts, water chestnuts, bamboo shoots, kale, red or green cabbage, bok choy, Chinese cabbage, green beans, zucchini, summer squash, eggplant, tomato.

Seasoning:
Asian style—A standard combination for an Asian style stir-fry is garlic, ginger, and tamari. Mince the garlic (2-4 cloves) and add it first to the oil before the vegetables. Stir on low heat to make sure it doesn't burn. After a minute or so, start adding veggies (more on that below). I don't like ginger fiber in food so I grate ginger, then squeeze it tightly in my fist and let the juice drip over the veggies about mid-way through the cooking. I sprinkle tamari on about the same time. Use 1-2 tablespoons grated ginger depending on how strong you want the flavor of ginger. Adjust tamari to taste, starting with about 2 tablespoons.

Variations: Use hot pepper oil as part of the oil; add a couple pieces of star anise to the oil after the garlic; add red pepper flakes; use ½ teaspoon Chinese Five Spice Powder.

Herbed—Use any combination of herbs, using a total of about 1½ teaspoons. Try basil, oregano, thyme, marjoram, rosemary, sage, or savory. Sauté garlic in olive oil to begin, as above.

Sauce: Vegetables release a fair amount of liquid as they cook. If you want a thicker sauce, add 1 or 1½ teaspoons arrowroot to 2 tablespoons of cold chicken or vegetable broth or cold water. Stir to dissolve. Clear a space in the veggies and pour mixture directly into liquid in skillet or wok. Bring heat to high and stir until sauce thickens and clears. Stir to coat vegetables.

Cooking: Use a large skillet or a wok over medium-high heat (a wok will cook things faster). Once garlic is browned, begin adding vegetables one at a time starting with the densest that take the longest to cook. Onions go first, carrots, broccoli, and cauliflower next, followed by celery and red or green cabbage and mushrooms. For Chinese cabbages and bok choy, separate leaves from stalk; stalks go in a minute or so before leaves. Sprouts, snow peas, mung sprouts, water chestnuts, bamboo shoots go in at the end just to heat slightly. Everything else goes somewhere in-between. Timing comes with practice! Strive for brightly colored, crisp-tender veggies.

SWEET AND SOUR RED CABBAGE
Serves 6

1½ pounds **Red Cabbage**, in thin slices
1 cup chopped **Onion**
2 **Tart Apples**, peeled, cored, and cut into bite-sized chunks
2 tablespoons **Raisins**
¼ cup **Cider Vinegar**
1 tablespoon **Olive Oil**
⅛ teaspoon **Allspice**
Salt to taste
3-5 drops **Stevia Liquid** or to taste

1.   Heat stock pot with oil. Add onions and sauté for 2 minutes. Add cabbage and stir to coat with oil. Add remaining ingredients except for stevia. Bring to a boil, cover, reduce heat, and simmer 30-45 minutes until cabbage is wilted and tender.

2.   Add stevia to bring sweetness to desired level.

1 serving = 97 kcal; 2g protein; 19g carbohydrate (4g fiber); 2.8g fat

SESAME-TAMARI WINTER SQUASH

Serves 8

If you've only had winter squash prepared with brown sugar, honey, or maple syrup, you're in for a nice surprise with this savory version. If you use an organic squash, don't be afraid to eat the nutritious skin, which will become tender and tasty as the squash bakes.

1 large, organic **Winter Squash** (Kabucha/Hokkaido, Butternut, Buttercup)
1 tablespoon **Sesame Oil**
4 tablespoons **Tamari**

1. Scrub skin of squash. Slice off stem end. Cut squash in half and thoroughly clean out all seeds and fibrous material. Cut in wedges or circles depending on type of squash.

2. Combine and blend the tamari and sesame oil. Using a pastry brush, paint all of the surfaces of the squash pieces, including the skin. You will not use all of the mixture. Store in a glass jar for later use. Place in a rectangular pan, cover with foil and bake at 375° for 30-40 minutes until squash pierces easily with a fork.

1 serving = 58 kcal; 2g protein; 12g carbohydrate (2g fiber); 0.9g unsaturated fat

FAUX MASHED POTATOES

Serves 4

Using roasted garlic and Neufchatel, I was able to successfully pass these off at Thanksgiving as the real thing to confirmed vegetable haters! It has now become a holiday standard at my house.

1 medium **Cauliflower**, cored and broken into florets (about 4 cups)
2 tablespoons **Half-and-Half**
2 teaspoons **Olive Oil**
Salt and Pepper to taste
Cooking Water as needed
4 tablespoons chopped **Scallions** for garnish (optional)

1. Bring salted water to boil, add cauliflower. After water returns to a boil, reduce heat to a simmer. Cook until florets can be easily pierced with a fork

2. Drain, reserving about a half-cup of the cooking water, and cool cauliflower slightly.

3. Place cauliflower in food processor or blender with olive oil and half-and-half, and blend until well puréed. Add small amounts of the cooking water if needed; be careful not to make the consistency too runny.

4. Season to taste with salt and pepper. Garnish with scallions if desired.

1 serving = 60 kcal; 2g protein; 5g carbohydrate (3g fiber); 3.8g unsaturated fat

---

Variations:
1. Add 2 ounces Neufchatel Cheese (a low-fat cream cheese) and/or 2 ounces grated low-fat cheddar.

2. Add 3-4 cloves roasted garlic and 2 ounces Neufchatel.

To roast garlic: Drizzle whole head of garlic with 1 teaspoon Olive Oil. Wrap head in foil and bake 45 minutes at 350°. Roasted garlic has a much milder and sweeter flavor than raw garlic and will keep for some time in the refrigerator.

With Neufchatel and Roasted Garlic: 95 kcal; 3g protein; 6g carbohydrate (3g fiber); 6.8g fat (2g saturated)

SIMPLE COLESLAW
Serves 4

½ head medium **Green Cabbage**, shredded
1 medium **Carrot,** shredded
¼ cup plain low-fat **Yogurt**
3 tablespoons **Mayonnaise**
2-3 tablespoons **Raw Cider Vinegar**
2 teaspoons **Celery Seed**
1 teaspoon **Dill Weed**
Salt and Pepper to taste

1. Remove core from cabbage, slice as thinly as possible vertically from top down through core end. Shred carrot using either food processor or grater.

2. Blend yogurt, mayonnaise, cider vinegar, celery seed, and dill weed.

3. Toss all ingredients together. Best if allowed to sit several hours to marinate. Season with salt and pepper to taste before serving.

1 cup = 56 kcal; 1g protein; 6g carbohydrate (1g fiber); 2.6g unsaturated fat

CREAMY BAKED STUFFED POTATOES

Serves 8

Potatoes are typically a high-glycemic food that can send your blood sugar skyward. As wonderful as they are, calorie for calorie they are not particularly nutrient dense, with the exception of potassium, in which they are very rich. If you are going to indulge, here's a delicious way to enjoy a baked potato that will temper the insulin-raising effect, add more nutrients, including essential fatty acids, and best of all, is a snap to prepare!

4 medium-sized organic **Baking Potatoes***
4 scoops **Unflavored Whey Protein Powder**
4 tablespoons **Flaxseed Oil**
½ cup chopped **Green Onion**
2 cups chopped, cooked **Broccoli**
    (can use **Kale, Collards, Zucchini** or other green veggies)
Salt and Pepper to taste

1. Preheat oven to 410°. Scrub potatoes, wrap individually in foil, and bake for 70 minutes.

2. Remove from oven, open foil and cut potatoes in half. Cool enough to handle. Scoop potato out of skin into a bowl, trying not to tear the skin.

3. Mix whey powder and flax oil into potato until creamy and well-blended. Add green onions and broccoli and stir to distribute throughout mixture. Add salt to taste.

4. Divide mixture between the 8 potato skins.

> * Baking potatoes can run quite large. A medium potato weighs 6-8 ounces.

One whole potato as prepared above makes a good small meal with a balance of protein, fat, and carbohydrate. Half a potato could be augmented with 2-3 ounces of additional protein and a salad, or some steamed veggies with 1-2 teaspoons of an olive oil and vinegar based dressing.

½ **baked, stuffed potato** = 187 kcal; 9g protein; 28g carbohydrate (3g fiber); 5.4 g unsaturated fat

CUCUMBER YOGURT SALAD

Serves 2

A cooling and refreshing side dish for hot weather or as a complement to spicy main dishes.

1 large **Cucumber**, peeled
¼ cup low-fat **Sour Cream**
2 tablespoons **Cider, Brown Rice, or White Wine Vinegar**
2 teaspoons **Dill Weed**
3-5 drops **Stevia Liquid**, to taste
Salt to taste

1. Run the tines of a fork lengthwise down the cucumber all the way around it. Cut it in half vertically, gently remove all seeds, and slice each half into ¼-inch slices. Place in bowl.

2. Add remaining ingredients to cucumber and toss gently to mix. Chill.

1 serving = 45 kcal; 2g protein; 9g carbohydrate (1g fiber); 0.2g saturated fat

GREEN BEANS, FENNEL, AND ONION

Serves 2

This is delicious when done on a grill, but is still good if done inside on the stovetop. If you've never tried fennel, it has a very mild licorice flavor that adds interest to an otherwise fairly ordinary vegetable dish.

½ pound fresh **Green String Beans**
2 stalks **Fennel**
½ medium **Onion** (cut whole onion in half vertically)
1 teaspoon **Olive Oil**
Juice of ½ **Lemon**
1 small clove **Garlic**, pressed
Salt and Pepper to taste

1. Wash beans and trim off stem end only. Lots of nutrients are in the other tip. Rinse each fennel stalk and slice into ¼-inch pieces. Place onion flat side down and cut into thin wedges.

2. Toss vegetables in a small bowl with olive oil, salt, and pepper.

3. When grill* is hot, place grill wok on top of grate. Add vegetables and cook for 10-12 minutes until vegetables are tender. While vegetables cook, combine lemon juice with garlic.

4. Before serving, toss with lemon juice and garlic or sprinkle over each serving. Adjust salt and pepper to taste.

1 serving = 82 kcal; 2g protein; 13g carbohydrate (2g fiber); 2.6g unsaturated fat

---

*This recipe can be done in a wok or frying pan on the stovetop. Instead of tossing vegetables with olive oil before cooking, put olive oil in skillet.

CREAMY CARROT AND PARSNIP
Serves 4-6

3 large **Carrots**
3 small-medium **Parsnips**
Pinch of **Salt**
Dash of **Olive Oil** (optional)

1. Scrub carrots and parsnips. Peel parsnips; if carrots are organic, leave peel on, otherwise peel them as well.

2. Cut each into uniform pieces, making parsnips a little bigger since they cook faster. Sprinkle with salt and let sit a few minutes to bring out sweetness.

3. Bring to boil about an inch and a half of water, add vegetables, and cook until they pierce easily with a fork (will depend on size of pieces, roughly 3-5 minutes).

4. Drain. Save cooking water for soup stock or mineral-rich, sweet drink.

5. Blend vegetables in blender or food processor until creamy. Add olive oil if desired.

½ **cup serving** = 52 kcal; 11g carbohydrate (3g fiber); 0.6g unsaturated fat

---

Variations: Try various combinations of root vegetables such as squash, carrot, and parsnip, or sweet potato (yam) and carrot.

Root vegetables (orange) are great sources of Vitamin A, satisfy your craving for sweet tastes, and energetically are grounding and nourishing.

CINNAMON ORANGE SQUASH
Serves 6

1 large **Winter Squash** or **Buttercup, Butternut,** or **Hokkaido**
6 tablespoons frozen **Orange Juice Concentrate**
2 teaspoons **Cinnamon**

1. Preheat oven to 375°. Wash the squash. Cut in half down from the stem end and scoop out all the seeds and membrane. Place orange juice concentrate in medium-sized bowl to soften.

2. Place halves, cut-side down on a cookie sheet with edges or in a baking dish. Add enough water to barely cover pan bottom.

3. Cover pan with foil and bake about 40 minutes until squash pierces easily with fork through skin. Remove from oven and allow to cool enough to handle.

4. Scoop squash from skin into bowl with orange juice concentrate. Add cinnamon and stir to distribute cinnamon and juice concentrate.

½ **cup serving** = 37 kcal; 9g carbohydrate (1g fiber); 2.6g unsaturated fat

To speed cooking time, slice each squash half into 5 or 6 wedges. Bake for 20-25 minutes. If you would like to serve squash wedges instead of mashed, do the following: Blend the OJ concentrate with 2 tablespoons water and the cinnamon in a blender. After cooking wedges 20-25 minutes, baste each with the mixture. Bake 5 minutes longer, uncovered.

BASIC BAKED YAM OR SWEET POTATO

Select yams or sweet potatoes that are firm, heavy, unwrinkled, and with relatively few blemishes. Scrub to clean, and trim the ends off if at all soft. Wrap each one in foil. Place in a 400° oven for 60-75 minutes until they're soft when squeezed. Cooking them at this higher temperature helps to bring out their natural sweetness.

> *A sweet potato or yam that is light-weight indicates it is old and dried out. Since they are harvested in the fall, this often happens to those that remain in summer, just before the new crop comes to market.

ROASTED CURRIED SWEET POTATOES
Serves 3-4

1 pound **Red Garnet Yams** (or other sweet potato), scrubbed and cubed into 1-inch pieces
1½ tablespoons **Butter** or **Olive Oil**
¾ teaspoon **Curry Powder**

1. Preheat oven to 450°. In a medium saucepan heat oil or butter and stir in curry powder.

2. Add potatoes and toss to coat well. Add salt and pepper if desired.

3. Place potatoes in baking pan. Roast in oven for 30 minutes until tender.

½ **cup serving with olive oil** = 166 kcal; 1g protein; 28g carbohydrate (4g fiber); 5.5g unsaturated fat

> *Any sweet potato or yam will work well, but I prefer the Red Garnet because of its sweetness. Red Garnets have a deep red/purple skin and tend to be longer and narrower than the yam usually seen in grocery stores. I have found that health food-type groceries are more likely to carry Red Garnets than regular grocery stores.

SWEET POTATO FRIES
Serves 2-3

1 medium to large **Red Garnet Yam (see page 303)**
1 teaspoon **Olive Oil** (spray bottle works well)
Salt to taste
Couple shakes **Cayenne Pepper** *or* 1 teaspoon **Cinnamon** (optional)

1. Scrub the skin of the yam; peel if not organic.

2. Slice into very thin slices. Place in bowl; spray or toss with olive oil to lightly
    coat all slices. Shake on cayenne or cinnamon, and a pinch or two of salt,
    and toss again.

3. Spread out potato slices on cookie sheet; bake at 375° for 20 minutes until
    soft or longer if you like them crisp. Turn slices over halfway through.

½ **cup serving** = 140 kcal; 1g protein; 28g carbohydrate (4g fiber);
0.1g unsaturated fat

Variation: To make a quicker, thicker fry, cut the yam in thirds, then cut each
third in half lengthwise. Flat side down, cut each piece into 3 or 4 wedge-
shaped slices. Follow step 3 above. These will be less crispy because of the
thickness but are also delicious. You can also broil instead of bake; if you
broil, watch more carefully so they don't get blackened.

PICKLED BEETS

Makes about 8 cups

From my friend Rachel Albert-Matesz of Next Generation Nutrition, this is a wonderful variation on the traditional sweet pickled beet.

3 pounds small- to medium-sized **Beets**, tops removed
2 **Bay Leaves**
Water

Marinade:
½ cup **Cider Vinegar**
1 tablespoon **Tamari**
⅛ teaspoon ground **Black Pepper**
1½ teaspoons **Dry Mustard**
1½ teaspoons ground **Cumin**

1. Wash beets thoroughly. Trim ends but do not peel or cut. In a 2-quart saucepan, place beets and bay leaves, with water to cover. Bring to a boil, then turn to simmer and cook about 30-60 minutes until beets can be pierced with knife tip (time will depend on beet size). While beets cook, mix marinade ingredients in medium-sized bowl.

2. Drain beets. Cut as desired, add to marinade and mix gently to coat. Let stand at least one hour before serving.

½ **cup serving** = 38 kcal; 1g protein; 8g carbohydrate (1g fiber); 0.1g unsaturated fat

GRAIN AND LEGUME
SIDE DISHES

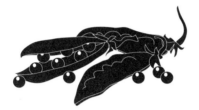

SARAH'S LENTIL SALAD

Serves 6

From weaver extraordinaire, Sarah Kaufmann. See her work at **www.sheshe.com/ kaufmann_studios/**

1 cup dry **Lentils**, rinsed
3 cups **Filtered Water**
1 cup **Carrots** diced small
⅔ cup diced **Red Onion**
½ cup chopped **Parsley**
2 cloves **Garlic**
¼ teaspoon **Worcestershire Sauce**
1 teaspoon **Salt**
¼ teaspoon ground **Black Pepper**

Dressing:
¼ cup **Olive Oil**
2 tablespoons **Red or Balsamic Wine Vinegar**
1 teaspoon **Dijon Mustard**
½ teaspoon **Oregano**

1. Place the lentils in a saucepan with water, salt, and garlic. Bring to a boil, reduce heat, and simmer 30-40 minutes until lentils are tender but still have some resistance when you bite into them. Drain off any excess water.

2. In a metal or nonreactive bowl, mix lentils with remaining seasoning, onions, parsley, and carrots.

3. In a small metal or ceramic bowl, whisk together dressing ingredients. Pour over lentil mixture and gently mix to coat. Tastes best if allowed to marinate a few hours before serving.

½ **cup serving** = 200 kcal; 9g protein; 21g carbohydrate (10g fiber); 9.4g fat (1g saturated)

---

*A **heat diffuser** is a flat metal plate with holes in it that allows heat through but keeps the pot from sitting directly on the heat. This prevents rice and other grains from sticking and scorching on the bottom of the pan.

WILD AND BROWN RICE MIX
Serves 8

1 cup short-grain **Brown Rice**
1 cup **Wild Rice**
3½ cups warm **Water**
1 teaspoon **Cider Vinegar**
1 teaspoon **Salt**

1. Rinse both rices thoroughly by swirling around in a bowl of water. Drain.

2. Place rice, warm water, and vinegar in a 2-quart saucepan the night before or morning of the day you plan to cook it. Soak for 8 or more hours.

3. Add salt. Cover. Bring to a boil. Place a heat diffuser* (*page 308) under the pot, turn down to a simmer. Simmer rice 45 to 50 minutes until soft and water is absorbed. Let sit 10 minutes then turn into bowl and fluff so steam can escape.

1 serving = 158 kcal; 4g protein; 33g carbohydrate (1g fiber); 0.9g unsaturated fat

---

Variations: Use leftover rice mixture to make Lentil and Rice Loaf on page 312. Or mix with some ground turkey, stuff into seeded red or green peppers, which you have parboiled for 3 minutes, and bake at 350° for 30 minutes. Add interest and fiber by throwing in any of the following: minced scallions; finely diced celery; chopped mushrooms; grated carrot; cooked, cut-up string beans; mung bean sprouts. Season with dried herbs and/or salsa, tomato sauce, or tamari.

Proper grain preparation: All grains contain antinutrient components—that is, they have naturally occurring substances that both inhibit digestion (enzyme inhibitors) and interfere with mineral absorption (phytates). All traditional cultures that used grains prepared them in ways that deactivated these antinutrient properties. Traditional cooking methods involve long slow cooking methods or preparations that allow fermentation to occur. In order to allow grains to enhance instead of deplete health, soaking of whole grains for an extended time in a slightly acidic liquid is suggested. For more information see the cookbook *Nourishing Traditions* by Sally Fallon or visit the website **www.westonaprice.org**

QUINOA TABOULI
Serves 8

1 cup **Quinoa**
1½ cups **Water**
Salt to taste
1 clove **Garlic**, pressed
4 cups chopped **Parsley**
3 tablespoons **Olive Oil**
Juice of 1 **Lemon**
1 medium **Cucumber**, seeded and diced (optional)

1. Rinse the quinoa in a fine mesh strainer. Place in pot with water and salt. Bring to boil, place a heat diffuser (see page 308) under the pot. Cover and simmer about 20 minutes until all the liquid is absorbed. Let it sit in covered pot off the heat another 10 minutes.

2. While the grain is cooking, rinse and chop parsley, discarding larger stems. Mix oil and lemon juice to taste and add pressed garlic. Place quinoa in wooden bowl and fluff with fork to help it cool.

3. Add the parsley to the grain and mix to evenly distribute. Add cucumbers if using, then add dressing to taste.

¾ **cup** = 98 kcal; 3g protein; 12g carbohydrate (2g fiber); 4.5g unsaturated fat

---

Variations: Add chopped meat such as chicken or turkey, and plenty of chopped vegetables, such as cooked broccoli, cauliflower, zucchini, or green beans, and raw vegetables, such as sweet peppers, carrots, scallions, radishes, cucumbers, or bok choy. Or try adding crumbled feta cheese.

BAKED BEANS
Serves 6

2 15-ounce cans **Great Northern Beans,** drained and rinsed
1 tablespoon **Ginger Juice,** squeezed from fresh grated **Ginger**
1 teaspoon dry **Mustard**
1½ tablespoons red or other dark **Miso**
½ cup **Water**
1 tablespoon **Molasses**
10 drops of **Stevia Liquid** (more to taste)

1. Mix together all but the beans, making sure miso is well blended into other liquids.

2. Stir liquid mixture into beans and bake in covered casserole at 350° until all the liquid is absorbed.

½ **cup** = 170 kcal; 10g protein; 30g carbohydrate (7g fiber); 0.8g unsaturated fat

LENTIL AND RICE LOAF
Serves 6

2 cups **cooked Lentils**
1 cup mixed **Wild and Brown Rice,** cooked (page 309)
½ cup chopped **Red or Green Bell Pepper**
½ cup chopped **Onion or Scallion**
1½ stalks **Celery,** diced
4 tablespoons **Tomato Paste**
¼ cup minced **Parsley**
2 tablespoons fresh **Basil** or 1½ teaspoons dry
2 tablespoons fresh **Oregano** or 1½ teaspoons dry
¼ teaspoon **Hot Red Pepper Flakes** (optional)
3 **Wasa Rye Crackers®** blended into crumbs
2 tablespoons **Sesame Tahini**
4 tablespoons hot **Water**

1. Combine all ingredients except sesame tahini and water in a bowl. Mix thoroughly.

2. Place 1 cup of above mixture into blender. Add sesame tahini and water. Blend until well-puréed. (You'll need to stop and move mixture around with a utensil.)

3. Blend puréed mixture with lentil-rice mixture in bowl. Spray or lightly wipe a loaf pan with olive oil. Turn mixture into pan.

4. Bake at 350° for 45 minutes.

1 serving = 176 kcal; 9g protein; 28g carbohydrate (2g fiber); 3.4g unsaturated fat

NUTRITION MAGICIAN'S 4-BEAN SALAD
Serves 5

1 15-ounce can **Westbrae® Salad Beans***, drained and rinsed
1 pound **Green Beans** (or use ½ pound each of waxed and green beans)
½ cup thinly sliced **Red Onion** (less if desired)
3 tablespoons **Apricot Preserves** (unsweetened, fruit only)
¼ cup **Cider Vinegar**

1. Trim vine end of green beans and cut beans into thirds. Steam until bright green and crisp tender, about 4-5 minutes. Remove from heat and drain.

2. In a medium-sized bowl, blend preserves and cider vinegar together until smooth.

3. Add green beans, canned beans, and onions to preserves mixture and stir to coat.

4. Cover and chill for several hours for flavors to meld.

1 cup serving = 81 kcal; 3g protein; 18g carbohydrate (3g fiber);
<1g unsaturated fat

---

*If this brand is not available to you, use an amount totaling 1½ cups (drained) from individual cans of kidney, garbanzo, and pinto beans.

POULTRY

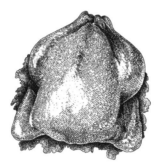

CHICKEN FOR A WEEK (PLUS STOCK)

This is a handy way to prepare food for a busy week ahead. Out of this you can have cold chicken for lunches, chicken salads, chicken soup, and meat for a casserole dish. Freeze whatever chicken you won't use in 3 days' time, in appropriately sized containers for later use.

2 **Fryer Chickens**, washed and excess fat cut off (about 5 pounds chicken)
1 package (4) **Chicken Backs,** washed and excess fat cut off
8 cups **Water**
1 large **Onion**, peeled and halved
4 stalks **Celery**, trimmed and cut into halves
1 **Carrot**, peeled
10 **Black Peppercorns**
2 **Bay Leaves**
2 **Garlic cloves**

1. Put chickens and vegetables in large soup pot with water and spices.

2. Bring to a boil, turn heat to simmer, cover, and cook one hour or until meat can easily be removed from bones. Remove chickens to a bowl to cool.

3. When cool enough to handle, remove meat from bones; discard skin. Add cleaned chicken bones and chicken backs to broth in soup pot and simmer covered another hour and a half. While soup simmers, divide chicken and put in containers. Freeze what you won't use in 3 days' time.

4. Strain broth. Discard vegetables and bones. Refrigerate soup overnight. Remove congealed fat from surface.

1 cup = 39 kcal; 4.9g protein; 0.9g carbohydrate; 1.1g fat (.4g saturated) (Nutrition analysis based on canned chicken stock; figures unavailable for homemade.)

HERB-ROASTED TURKEY BREAST

This is easy to make and a good source of protein to have around for the week. Most recipes for turkey use too high a temperature, causing the turkey meat to become dried out and unappealing. This slow, low-heat roasting will give you meat that is moist.

2½ to 3 pounds **Turkey Breast** (bone-in or boneless)
2 tablespoons **Olive Oil**
1 large clove **Garlic**, crushed
1 teaspoon **Sage**
½ teaspoon **Thyme**
1 teaspoon **Marjoram**
½ teaspoon **Salt**
1 teaspoon **Black Pepper**

1. Rinse turkey breast and pat dry. Place in small roasting pan. Preheat oven to 425°.

2. Heat olive oil in small sauté pan. Add garlic and stir to keep from browning, about a minute. Add other herbs and sauté 2 minutes. Remove from heat.

3. Spread herb mixture all over turkey breast, pushing some under skin. Add ½ cup water to bottom of pan or enough to cover pan with about ¼ inch of water.

4. Roast at 425° for 15 minutes. Turn heat to 325° and roast for 45-55 minutes more for boneless, 50-60 for bone-in. Turkey will continue to cook from internal heat after it's removed from oven.

5. Cool before slicing. Freeze packages of cooked turkey if desired.

4 ounces with skin* = 244 kcal; 32g protein; 11.7g fat (2g saturated)
4 ounces without skin = 125 kcal; 32g protein; 2g fat (1g saturated)

> *Poultry skin contains very little saturated fat, so there is no need to avoid it if you like it. Just be sure to limit fat intake somewhere else to balance your day's intake.

TURKEY BLACK BEAN SALAD WITH CHILI-LIME DRESSING
Serves 5

12 ounces **Roasted Turkey Breast**, diced (page 317)
1 cup canned **Black Beans**, drained and rinsed
1 **Avocado**, diced
1½ cup **Cherry Tomatoes**
½ cup thinly sliced **Scallions**
1½ cups diced **Jicama**
8 cups bite-sized **Romaine Lettuce**
6 tablespoons **Chili-Lime Dressing** (below)

1. Combine first 6 ingredients in a medium-sized bowl. Add dressing and toss to mix thoroughly.

2. Serve on individual plates on bed of romaine leaves.

Chili-Lime Dressing

¼ cup fresh **Lime Juice**
1⅓ teaspoons **Cider Vinegar**
½ teaspoon **Chili Powder**
¼ teaspoon **Cumin**
¼ cup **Olive Oil**
1 medium clove **Garlic**, crushed
1 medium **Anaheim Chili Pepper**, roasted, peeled, seeded, and chopped*

1. Roast pepper by placing under broiler or holding over gas flame and allowing skin to char. Turn so that entire pepper is blackened. Place in brown paper bag to cool. When pepper is cool enough to handle, peel skin off and remove seeds.

2. Combine dressing ingredients in blender and blend until smooth.

1 serving = 332 kcal; 26g protein; 21g carbohydrate (8g fiber); 16.7g fat (2g saturated)

---

* Wear rubber gloves whenever cutting up chili peppers. Most of the hot oils that irritate skin and eyes are in the membranes that you cut out and discard.

ITALIAN TURKEY SAUSAGE & TOMATO STEW
Serves 8

Since the best diet for beating weight gain, depression, diabetes, heart disease, and fatigue limits simple carbohydrates, including pasta, I made this recipe to be enjoyed as a hearty soup with a sprinkling of Parmesan cheese. You'll almost always find this in my freezer from October to May!

1 tablespoon **Olive Oil**
3 large cloves **Garlic,** finely chopped
2 cup coarsely chopped **Onions** (approximately 1 large, 2 small)
2 pounds **Italian Turkey Sausage** (hot or mild according to preference)
2 ribs **Celery**, thinly sliced
1 large **Carrot**, finely chopped
3 28-ounce cans **Diced Tomatoes**, including juice
¼ cup **Tomato Paste**
2 teaspoons dried **Oregano**
¼ teaspoon dried ground **Rosemary** or 1 teaspoon dried leaves
¾ teaspoons ground **Fennel**
2 **Bay Leaves**
½ teaspoon **Salt** or to taste
Freshly ground **Black Pepper** to taste
Parmesan Cheese (optional)

1. Prepare vegetables. Remove sausage from casings if necessary. Heat a large stock pot over medium heat, and when hot, add oil.

2. Sauté garlic and onion over low heat, stirring frequently for 3 minutes. Add sausage. Stir to break into small pieces and brown thoroughly.

3. Add remaining ingredients and stir well, scraping up any browned goodies sticking to bottom of pot. Bring to a boil, reduce heat, and simmer covered for 40 minutes.

4. Remove bay leaves and season to taste with salt and pepper. Cool to room temperature and refrigerate or freeze if desired.

1½ cups = 268 kcal; 23g protein; 14g carbohydrate (3g fiber); 11.3g fat (2g saturated)
1 tablespoon grated Parmesan = 23 kcal; 2g protein; 2g fat (1g saturated)

SIMPLE CHICKEN AND CHICKPEA STIR-FRY

Serves 4

1 pound **Boneless Chicken Breast**
1 cup cooked **Chickpeas** (garbanzo beans), liquid saved
2 medium **Onions**
1 large **Carrot**
1 pound **Mushrooms**, sliced
4 teaspoons **Olive Oil**
1 tablespoon **Tamari** or to taste

1. Wash chicken; pat dry. Cut each breast in half lengthwise and slice into ¼-
    to ½-inch slices.*

2. Cut onions in half through root end and peel. Cut each half in half horizon-
    tally. Cut half-moon slices. Slice carrot in half lengthwise. Placing flat side
    down, slice each half thinly on a diagonal.

3. Heat cast iron skillet. Add oil when hot, then add onions and stir for 2
    minutes. Add carrot slices and sauté a minute more. Add mushrooms; stir
    to coat with oil. Add tamari, chicken pieces, and chickpeas. Stir over
    medium heat for 10 minutes until chicken is done through. Add liquid from
    chickpeas as needed while cooking to keep mixture from becoming too dry.

1 serving = 311 kcal; 29g protein; 28g carbohydrate (5g fiber); 9.2g fat (1g saturated)

---

*If you can work with the chicken when it is still slightly frozen, it is much
easier to slice.

TURKEY CHILI

Serves 4-6

Using several types of chili pepper gives the chili a more interesting and complex flavor. Feel free to experiment to get a dish that's more than just spicy tomato sauce! Chili is best made a day in advance to give flavors time to develop. Chili freezes very well. Vegetarians can easily substitute tempeh for the meat.

1 pound **Ground Turkey** (light, dark, or a mixture) or 1 pound **Tempeh*** (page 324)
2 cups chopped **Onion**
2 stalks **Celery**, thinly sliced
1 15-ounce can **Kidney Beans**, drained and rinsed
1 28-ounce can **Peeled, Ground, or Chopped Tomatoes**
1 large clove **Garlic**, minced
2 teaspoons **Olive Oil**
1½ teaspoons **Cumin**
2 tablespoons **Chili Powder**
1 teaspoon **Salt** or to taste
2 dried **Chipotle Chilies** (optional), soaked in hot water 10 minutes
½ teaspoon **Red Pepper Flakes** (optional)

1. Heat a 4-quart soup or stockpot. Add oil and spread around to coat pan. Immediately add chopped onions and garlic and stir frequently for 2-3 minutes on medium-low heat.

2. Add sliced celery; sauté for another 2 minutes.

3. Add ground turkey and stir to break up. Sauté for about 5 minutes until turkey starts to lose pink color. Add spices and continue cooking and stirring another couple minutes.

4. Add tomatoes, chipotle chili if using, and beans. Bring to boil, reduce heat, cover, and simmer 20 minutes on low.

1 cup = 228 kcal; 20g protein; 22g carbohydrate (3g fiber); 7.1g fat
(2g saturated)
Fat content will vary depending on use of light or dark meat. This analysis was based on 1 pound of dark meat, turkey.

MEATBALLS FOR BLUE CHEESE FANS
Makes 34 meatballs
A nice change from ordinary meatballs.

¾ pound **Ground Turkey Dark Meat**
¾ pound **Ground Turkey Breast**
1 **Egg or 2 Whites**
2 ounces **Blue Cheese**
2 teaspoons dried **Sage Leaves** (or ¾-1 teaspoon powder)
2 cloves **Garlic,** crushed
½ teaspoon **Black Pepper**
½ teaspoon **Salt**
¾ cup minced fresh **Parsley**

1. In a medium-sized mixing bowl, combine all ingredients and mix to blend well. With wet hands, form into small (1-inch diameter) meatballs. You should get about 34 balls.

2. Place on baking sheet and bake at 350° for 15-20 minutes until no longer pink in center. Or, if you have some chicken, turkey, or light vegetable stock available, simmer the meatballs in stock, on low heat, with cover for same amount of time.

Each meatball = 35 kcal; 4g protein; 1.7g fat (.6g saturated)

TURKEY TOSS FOR TWO
Serves 2

In a small bowl, mix together:

8-10 ounces **Herb Roasted Turkey Breast** (page 317) skin removed and cubed
6 tablespoons (roughly ⅔) **Avocado**, diced
½ cup thinly sliced **Red Onion**
1 cup **Artichoke Hearts**, drained
4 tablespoons **Mustard Apple Vinaigrette** (page 265)

1 serving = 328 kcal; 28 g protein; 13g carbohydrate (4g fiber); 18.6g fat (3g saturated)

CHICKEN OR TEMPEH FAJITAS
Serves 4

1 pound boneless, skinless **Chicken Breast or** 2 8-ounce packages **Tempeh***
1 cups sliced **Onions** (about 1 medium)
2 cups sliced **Red Bell Pepper**
2 cups sliced **Green Bell Pepper**
2 cups sliced **Mushrooms**
1 teaspoon **Chili Powder**
½ teaspoon **Cumin**
¼ teaspoon **Red Pepper Flakes** (or to taste)
Salt and Pepper to taste
½ cup mashed **Avocado**
½ cup low-fat **Sour Cream**
2 teaspoons **Olive Oil**
½ cup mild or medium **Salsa** (optional)

1. Heat cast iron skillet or large frying pan. When hot, add olive oil. Add sliced onion and stir to coat evenly with oil. Sauté for 2-3 minutes on medium-low heat, stirring frequently.

2. If you will be using tempeh, cut the tempeh into ½-inch x 1-inch pieces and place in a covered steamer basket over simmering water for 10 minutes.

3. Add peppers to the onions and stir for a minute or two, then add mushrooms and sauté for another minute or two.

4. Add chicken or steamed tempeh pieces and stir to mix. Add spices and allow to simmer on low heat until vegetables are tender and chicken or tofu is cooked through, about 15 minutes.

5. Serve with salsa, avocado, and low-fat sour cream if desired.

1 serving (chicken) = 297 kcal; 29g protein; 19g carbohydrate (3g fiber); 12.6g fat (2g saturated)
1 serving (tempeh) = 337 kcal; 21g protein; 34g carbohydrate (3g fiber); 15.4g fat (2g saturated)
Nutritional counts include 2 tablespoons each: salsa, avocado, and low-fat sour cream.

Variations: Boneless chicken or tempeh could be replaced with ground turkey or ground chicken or lean ground beef, sirloin, eye of round, or other lean cut. If you use a cut of meat with significantly more saturated fat than chicken white meat, you can, if you want, reduce fat somewhere else in recipe or meal (e.g., avocado, sour cream, or olive oil—or try using the salsa to sauté instead of the oil).

*Tempeh is a pressed cake of cooked, fermented soybeans, often with the addition of various grains. It has a nutty flavor and absorbs the flavors of marinades and sauces very well. Steam tempeh for 10 minutes over simmering water in a covered pot, before adding to any recipe.

CRISPY SESAME FINGERS

Serves 5
Want a healthful version of a fast-food chicken nugget? Try this with turkey or boneless chicken pieces!

1 pound **Turkey Tenderloins**, cut into 1-inch x 2-inch strips
½ cup plus 2 tablespoons **Dried Onion Flakes**
½ cup plus 2 tablespoons **Sesame Seeds**
¼ teaspoon **Salt**
¼ teaspoon **Black Pepper**
1 **Egg White**, beaten
4 teaspoons **Olive Oil**, divided

1. In a small bowl mix together onion flakes, sesame seeds, salt, and pepper.

2. Heat heavy-bottomed skillet. Begin dipping turkey strips in egg white then in sesame mixture. When frying pan is hot, add 2 teaspoons oil and spread around pan. Place coated turkey strips in hot pan and cook for 2-3 minutes. Turn over and cook 2-3 minutes on other side. You should be able to do 2 batches (about ½ the recipe) before needing to add the remaining oil.

1 serving = 259 kcal; 27g protein; 9g carbohydrate (1g fiber); 13.6g unsaturated fat

SPECKLED CHICKEN PATTIES
Serves 4

1 pound boneless, skinless **Chicken Breast,** ground
1 clove **Garlic**, pressed
1 teaspoon **Salt**
½ teaspoon **White Pepper**
½ teaspoon **Cumin**
½ teaspoon **Paprika**
3 tablespoons finely diced **Green Bell Pepper**
3 tablespoons finely diced **Red Bell Pepper**
3 tablespoons minced **Parsley**
2 teaspoons **Olive Oil**

1. Mix all ingredients until well combined. Form into 4 patties.

2. Heat cast iron or heavy skillet until hot, then add olive oil. Sauté chicken patties 3-5 minutes per side until cooked through.

1 patty = 152 kcal; 24g protein; 1g carbohydrate; 6g fat (1g saturated)

QUICK THAI CHICKEN
Serves 4

The trick to making ethnic recipes quick and easy is having the "unusual" ingredients already in your pantry.

1½ pounds **Boneless Chicken Breast**
1 **Red Bell Pepper**, sliced
1 **Green Bell Pepper**, sliced
1 medium **Onion**, sliced
1½-inch piece **Ginger Root**
1 large clove **Garlic**
1 tablespoon minced **Lemon Grass** (about 3 inches)
1 3- to 4-inch **Hot Red Finger Pepper**
1 tablespoon **Fish Sauce** (available in Asian food market or ethnic section of grocery)
1 tablespoon **Peanut Oil**
½ cup **Lite Coconut Milk**
¼ teaspoon **Red Curry Paste** (available as with fish sauce)
Pinch or two of **Salt**

1. Remove seeds from hot red pepper. Be sure to wear rubber gloves while handling. Mince the garlic, ginger, and hot red pepper by hand or in mini food processor. Separately, mince the lemon grass and set aside. Cut chicken breasts in half and slice halves into ½-inch slices.

2. Heat cast iron or other skillet. When hot, add peanut oil. Add ginger, garlic, pepper mixture and sauté and stir for 1-2 minutes on medium heat.

3. Add onions and sauté another 2 minutes, stirring occasionally. Add peppers and minced lemon grass pieces and stir to coat with oil. Sauté for a minute or two before adding chicken pieces and fish sauce.

4. Allow chicken and vegetable to cook on medium-low heat for about 10-12 minutes, stirring frequently until chicken pieces appear white and firm. Pour coconut milk into pan and add curry paste, stirring to mix into juices.

1 serving = 246 kcal; 31g protein; 8g carbohydrate (1g fiber); 9.7g fat (2g saturated)

INDOOR BARBECUED CHICKEN

Serves 5

Although eating chicken skin has become a dietary heresy, an occasional indulgence, if you like it, in this mostly unsaturated fat, is fine. Simply balance out your fat intake over the rest of that day or the next. And if you don't care to indulge, try the boneless breast variation below.

2 to 2½ pounds cut-up **Fryer Chicken**, rinsed and patted dry
¾ cup **Nutrition Magician's Barbecue Sauce** (page 267)
Salt and pepper

1. Salt and pepper the chicken pieces and place in broiling pan. Broil pieces about 20 minutes until chicken is white and juices lose their pink color. Turn pieces over once, midway through cooking.

2. Remove chicken from oven. Use a spoon to spread 2 tablespoons BBQ sauce over each piece. Return to broiler and broil another 3-4 minutes until sauce starts to brown.

⅕ **chicken** = 356 kcal; 38g protein; 5g carbohydrate; 18.9g fat (5g saturated)

Variation (Serves 4)
1¼ pounds boneless, skinless **Chicken Breast**
½ cup **Nutriton Magician's Barbecue Sauce** (page 267)
1 **Sweet Red Bell Pepper**, in strips
1 **Green Bell Pepper**, in strips
1 medium **Onion**, in thin wedges
¼ to ½ cup **Chicken Stock**
2 teaspoons **Olive Oil**

1. In large skillet, heat olive oil. Add onions and sauté for 4-5 minutes, stirring periodically.

2. Add red and green pepper strips and continue sautéing and stirring until peppers soften. While vegetables cook, cut chicken into small strips.

3. Add barbecue sauce and ¼ cup stock to onions and peppers; add chicken pieces. Simmer over low to medium heat until chicken pieces are cooked through, about 10-12 minutes. Add extra stock as necessary while cooking to keep BBQ sauce from getting too thick and sticking to pan.

1 serving = 241 kcal; 26g protein; 12g carbohydrate; 8g fat (1g saturated)

ROMAINE ROLL-UPS

Serves 2-4

Stumped by the thought of lunch without a sandwich? Try these dandy rolls in a packed lunch or for a snack.

8 leaves **Romaine* or Bibb Lettuce**, rinsed and dried
10 ounces sliced deli **Turkey**
½ cup prepared **Hummus** (available in many grocery stores)
6 tablespoons mashed **Avocado**

1. For each roll, place two lettuce leaves so they overlap but are not directly on top of each other.

2. Lay ¼ of the turkey slices on top of lettuce. Spread 2 tablespoons hummus followed by 1½ tablespoons avocado. Gently roll up burrito style.

1 roll = 146 kcal; 14.5g protein; 9g carbohydrate (3g fiber); 5.9g fat

---

*If you use Romaine lettuce, cut off lowest part of leaf where stem is thick, so leaf can roll up.

Variation: Sprinkle with chopped scallions, finely diced sweet red bell peppers, shredded carrots, or alfalfa sprouts.

GRILLED TURKEY KOFTAS

Serves 4

Koftas are a Mediterranean grilled specialty, traditionally using beef or lamb.

1 pound **Ground Turkey***
⅓ cup finely diced **Sweet Red Bell Pepper**
4 pieces **Sun-Dried Tomato**, finely chopped
1 tablespoon fresh **Oregano** or 1 teaspoon dried
1 tablespoon fresh **Basil** or 1 teaspoon dried
1 teaspoon fresh **Thyme** or ¼ teaspoon dried
½ teaspoon **Salt**
½ teaspoon ground **Black Pepper**
Oil from Sun-Dried Tomatoes or Olive Oil for brushing
4 **Wooden Skewers** soaked 5 minutes in water

1. Place all ingredients except oil in small mixing bowl and mix with hands until well-combined.

2. To form koftas, run hands under cold water to keep meat from sticking. Divide mixture into 4 portions. For each portion, press and roll into sausage shape. Put skewer through middle. Using both a pressing and a stretching motion, extend sausage roll along length of skewer leaving about 1½ inches at thick end of skewer for handling on grill. Slightly flatten kofta. Place on plate. If not grilling immediately, cover and refrigerate.

3. To grill, brush top of koftas with oil, place oil side down on grill grate. Grill 3-4 minutes, brush tops with oil, turn, and grill 3-4 minutes on other side to finish.

1 kofta (light ground) = 152 kcal; 26g protein; 1g carbohydrate; 4.3g unsaturated fat
1 kofta (dark ground) = 202 kcal; 20g protein; 1g carbohydrate; 12.2g fat (2g saturated)

Variation: An alternative way to prepare this without the grill would be to bake or broil. Or try making walnut-sized meatballs from the mixture and simmering for about twenty minutes in ½ cup of a good tomato sauce mixed with ½ cup water. Cooked koftas and meatballs keep well in freezer for 2-3 months.

*Using white meat turkey will give a leaner dish; however, dark meat poultry provides a lot of zinc, a mineral we often lack, that helps with immunity, wound healing, vision, smell and taste, and male sexual function. So alternating use of light and dark meat poultry is good for your health, even with the additional (mostly unsaturated) fat contained in dark meat poultry.

LEMON ROSEMARY CHICKEN

Serves 4

This is an especially simple preparation that gives a refreshing taste to the chicken. I like this recipe in hotter weather. It can easily be doubled or tripled for a crowd or for the freezer.

4 split **Chicken Breasts**
Juice of 3 **Lemons**
3 large cloves **Garlic**, minced
½ teaspoon **Rosemary** (powdered) or 1 teaspoon crushed if whole

1. Combine lemon juice, rosemary, and garlic.

2. Pour over chicken pieces in flat container. Cover and refrigerate for 2 or more hours.

3. Bake at 350° for 20-25 minutes until cooked through. Chicken can also be broiled, skin-side up, for approximately same amount of time, depending on distance from flame.

1 split breast (approximately 5 ounces) = 249 kcal; 30.2g protein; 13.4g fat (3.8g saturated)

> **Variation:** Use boneless breast or boneless thigh pieces. Do not broil boneless breast or chicken will become dry and tough.

SIMPLE CHICKEN SALAD
Serves 2

6-8 ounces shredded or bite-sized cooked **Chicken Breast**
   (use lower amount with variation #1)
1 stalk **Celery**, finely diced
1 **Scallion**, minced
3 tablespoons **Spectrum® Light Mayonnaise**
Salt and Pepper to taste
½ **Green Bell Pepper**, seeded and diced (optional)

Combine all ingredients in a small bowl.

1 serving = 190 kcal; 24g protein; 3g carbohydrate; 8.2g unsaturated fat

---

Variations: Follow main recipe, making the changes below:

#1 Add:
   2 pieces crisp **Bacon**, crumbled
   1 **Hard-Boiled Egg**, mashed
   1 teaspoon **Celery Seed**
   Pinch **Cayenne Pepper**
   (use only 6 ounces cooked chicken)

1 serving = 232 kcal; 24g protein; 4g carbohydrate; 12.6g fat (2g saturated)

#2 Omit green pepper and add:
   ½ cup seedless **Grapes,** cut in half; or 1 **Mango**, peeled and cubed
   Squeeze of fresh **Lime Juice**
   ¼ cup fresh **Cilantro**
   1 teaspoon of **Curry Powder** (optional)

1 serving (with mango) = 257 kcal; 24g protein; 20g carbohydrate
(2g fiber); 8.5g unsaturated fat
(with grapes) = 204 kcal; 24g protein;7g carbohydrate; 8.3g unsaturated fat

ITALIAN SAUSAGE, CABBAGE, AND KRAUT
Serves 4

1 pound **Italian Turkey Sausage** (hot, mild, or a combination)
6 cups sliced **Cabbage** (small head, about 1½ pounds)
3 cups fresh **Sauerkraut***
1 small **Onion**, sliced in half moons
1½ tablespoons **Olive Oil**
1 medium **Red Bell Pepper**, seeded and diced
2 tablespoons **Dijon Mustard**
¼ cup **Water**

1. Heat a large cast iron or other heavy skillet on medium. Add oil. When hot, add cabbage and stir to coat with oil. Sauté cabbage, stirring periodically, for about 5 minutes.

2. While cabbage cooks, drain sauerkraut. If too salty, rinse and drain well. Add drained kraut to cabbage. Add diced peppers. Stir and sauté another 5 minutes.

3. Slice or break up Italian sausage. Add to skillet. Turn so sausage pieces can brown on bottom of skillet. When browned, stir everything together, cover skillet, and reduce heat slightly. Cook for 15 minutes or until sausage is cooked through.

4. Blend Dijon mustard with water. Pour over sausage, cabbage, and kraut. Stir to blend and simmer a couple minutes more. Add more mustard diluted with a little water if you like a stronger flavor.

1 serving = 303 kcal; 22g protein; 17g carbohydrate (8g fiber); 15.1g fat (3g saturated)

*Fresh Sauerkraut can be found in bags in refrigerator cases in the grocery. Usually it is kept with the hot dog/sausage-type items.

CABBAGE LASAGNA

Serves 6

Miss that pasta? This recipe takes a bit more fussing but the result is worth it and can be used for several meals. You'll get all the good tastes of lasagna without the heaviness and blood sugar rise of the lasagna noodles.

1 medium to large **Green Cabbage**
1 tablespoon **Olive Oil**
2 cloves **Garlic**, minced
1 **Green Bell Pepper**, diced
1 cup diced **Onion**
1 pound **Lean Ground Turkey**
1½ cups prepared **Tomato Sauce**
1 teaspoon **Oregano**
1 teaspoon **Basil**
½ teaspoon **Salt**
1 teaspoon **Black Pepper**
1 cup grated low-fat **Mozzarella Cheese**
1 cup low-fat **Cottage or Ricotta Cheese**
½ cup grated **Parmesan Cheese**

1. Wash cabbage and remove tough outer leaves. Remove core of cabbage with sharp paring knife until you can peel off 12 individual leaves. Bring large pot of water to a boil. Drop half the leaves into water and let simmer for 5 minutes, or until leaves are tender but not mushy. Remove and drain leaves. Repeat this process with remaining leaves.

2. Heat cast iron or other heavy skillet. When hot add oil, onions and minced garlic. Stir for 2-3 minutes.

3. Add green pepper and sauté 3 minutes more or until onions are translucent and peppers softened. Then add ground turkey, stir to break up and sauté for 10-12 minutes more.

4. Add tomato sauce and spices and mix to combine well; simmer 5 minutes to let flavors blend.

5. Spray a 9-inch x 13-inch lasagna pan with olive oil. Line bottom of pan with a layer of cabbage leaves. Top with half of sauce mixture. Add ⅓ of grated mozzarella and ½ of cottage or ricotta cheese.

6. Add second layer of cabbage leaves. Repeat sauce and cheeses. Top with remaining ⅓ of mozzarella and sprinkle with Parmesan.

7. Bake at 350° covered, for 20 minutes. Uncover and bake 5 minutes more. Let sit 10 minutes before serving.

1 serving = 284 kcal ; 31g protein; 13g carbohydrate (2g fiber); 10.4g fat (4g saturated)

ROCKY'S MAMA'S TURKEY MEATLOAF

Serves 6-9

Rocky, my Sharpei, has unfortunately never tasted this meatloaf, because he's allergic to turkey among dozens of other foods. But you can enjoy it! This freezes very well, so while you're at it, make two and freeze one for later.

1½ pounds **Ground Turkey**
6 **Egg Whites** (can reconstitute from powder—see page 255)
1 cup **Rolled Oats**
¾ cup chopped **Green Bell Pepper**
1½ cups chopped **Mushrooms**
1 tablespoon **Tamari**
2 cloves **Garlic,** crushed, or 1 teaspoon **Garlic Powder**
1 teaspoon **Oregano**
½ teaspoon **Sage**
½ teaspoon **Salt**
½ teaspoon **Black Pepper**

1. Preheat oven to 425°. Mix everything together in a mixing bowl until well-blended.

2. Use an oil spray bottle if available to lightly coat a loaf pan; otherwise use waxed paper with small amount of oil.

3. Press meat into loaf pan. Bake for 15 minutes at 425°, then turn down heat to 350° and bake for 35 minutes more. Allow to cool 10-15 minutes before removing from pan or slicing. Slice into 9 slices.

1 slice = 198 kcal; 18g protein; 12g carbohydrate; 7.6g fat (1g saturated)

INDIAN MEATBALLS WITH FRESH YOGURT-CILANTRO SAUCE
Serves 5

1¼ pounds **Ground Chicken Breast**
2 teaspoons **Olive Oil**
½ small **Jalapeño Pepper**
Pinch to ⅛ teaspoon **Cayenne Pepper**
1 teaspoon **Cumin Seed**
1 teaspoon **Ground Coriander**
1 teaspoon **Ground Ginger**
½ teaspoon **Salt**
¼ - ½ cup **Water**

1. Wearing rubber gloves, seed and mince jalapeño pepper.

2. In small skillet, heat olive oil. Add cumin seed and stir until it begins to crackle and turn brown. Add remaining spices except for salt and stir over low heat for a minute more.

3. Add oil and spice mixture along with salt to ground chicken. Mix thoroughly. Form into balls about the size of a jumbo olive, making about 30.

4. Place meatballs in large pot and add enough water to cover bottom of pan. Simmer covered for 15 minutes until meatballs are cooked through.

5. Serve with Yogurt-Cilantro Sauce below.

Yogurt-Cilantro Sauce (Serves 4)

1 cup plain, low-fat **Yogurt**
½ cup minced, fresh **Cilantro**
2-inch piece fresh **Ginger Root, grated**
1 teaspoon fresh **Lemon Juice**

1. Place ⅓ cup yogurt and cilantro in blender. Blend until smooth. Place in bowl.

2. Holding ginger gratings in your fist over the yogurt bowl, squeeze juice out of fiber. Add lemon juice. Blend into yogurt mixture. Flavors develop if sauce has a chance to chill.

1 serving meatballs with sauce = 176 kcal; 26g protein; 4g carbohydrate; 6.2g fat (1g saturated)

BEEF, LAMB, AND PORK

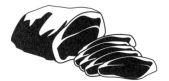

MEDITERRANEAN MEATLOAF
Serves 9

1½ pounds **Ground Sirloin**
2 **Egg Whites**
⅔ cup **Rolled Oats**
2 cloves **Garlic**, crushed
1 teaspoon **Olive Oil**
2 **Green Onions**, thinly sliced, whites and greens
1 stalk **Celery**, diced
10 **Kalamata Olives**, pitted and chopped
¼ cup fresh **Parsley** (or 2 tablespoons dried)
1 tablespoon **Oregano** flakes (or 1½ teaspoons ground)

1. Preheat oven to 350°. Sauté garlic in oil for a minute or two until lightly browned.

2. Combine all ingredients in a mixing bowl, including sautéed garlic, but leave oil out. Mix until everything is well-incorporated.

3. Use leftover oil from garlic to oil a loaf pan. Press meat into pan; bake 45 minutes or until liquid from meat runs clear. Cool before slicing.

1 serving = 186 kcal; 16g protein; 4g carbohydrate; 10.7g fat (3g saturated)

> **Variation:** Use ground turkey instead of ground sirloin.
> **1 serving with lean turkey** = 119 kcal; 19g protein; 4g carbohydrate; 2.4g unsaturated fat
> **1 serving with dark turkey** = 152 kcal; 15g protein; 4g carbohydrate; 7.7g fat (1g saturated)

LAMB AND ZUCCHINI MEATBALLS
Makes 18-20 meatballs

1 pound lean **Ground Lamb**
2 **Wasa® Crackers**, blended into fine crumbs
1 medium **Zucchini**, grated and squeezed of excess liquid
2 **Egg Whites**
¼ cup **Chunky, Fat-Free Tomato Sauce**
2 cloves **Garlic**, crushed or minced finely
2 tablespoons chopped fresh **Parsley**
1 teaspoon **Oregano**
½ teaspoon ground **Rosemary**
⅜ teaspoon **Salt**

1. Combine all ingredients in medium mixing bowl until well-blended. Form into 18-20 small balls. Place on cookie sheet that has been lightly sprayed with oil.

2. Bake at 425° for 10 minutes. Turn balls and cook another 5 minutes.

1 meatball = 63 kcal; 5g protein; 1g carbohydrate; 2.9g fat (1g saturated)

SPICY MEATBALL MAMBO
Makes 15 meatballs

1 pound lean **Ground Beef** (10% or less fat)
¼ cup diced **Red Onion**
2 stalks **Celery,** sliced
1 **Red Bell Pepper**, seeded and chopped
2 dried **Chipotle Peppers***
1 medium **Zucchini**, cut in half moons
1 cup prepared **Pasta Sauce** (meatless)
½ cup **Salsa**
1 cup **water**
¾ teaspoon ground **Cumin**
¼ teaspoon **Red Pepper Flakes**
¼ teaspoon **Salt** or to taste

1. Soak chipotle in hot water 10 minutes, then remove, discarding water.

2. In heavy-bottomed pot, stir pasta sauce, salsa, and water together. Add celery, red peppers, and chipotle peppers. Bring to a boil, then turn heat down to a simmer.

3. While vegetables are cooking, mix ground beef with diced red onion, salt, red pepper flakes, and cumin. Form into meatballs about the size of a walnut in a shell; you should get about 15.

4. Add meatballs to sauce and simmer with lid on for 15 minutes. Remove lid and add zucchini, letting it sit on top. Simmer five minutes more until zucchini is tender but not mushy. Stir together and adjust seasoning to taste.

1 meatball with ¼ cup sauce = 76 kcal; 4g protein; 3g carbohydrate; 4g fat (1g saturated)

*Chipotle peppers are a type of chili pepper that has been dried and smoked. Along with adding some heat to a dish as any other hot pepper would, it also gives the same kind of smoky flavor that liquid smoke or cooking with a ham hock gives.

SWEET 'N' SOUR PORK WITH NAPPA CABBAGE

Serves 4

Don't be put off by the need to make the dressing in order to complete this recipe. The sweet and tangy dressing can be made ahead and keeps well in the refrigerator. And, it's a snap to make.

1 pound **Pork Loin**, trimmed of fat, cut into strips ¼-inch x 1½-inches
10 cups sliced **Nappa Cabbage**, rinsed
1 large **Onion**, sliced in thin wedges
1 large **Red Bell Pepper**, thinly sliced
1 small can sliced **Water Chestnuts**, drained
1 cup **Southeast Asian Sesame Pineapple Dressing** (recipe on following page)
2 teaspoons **Arrowroot** dissolved in 1 tablespoon cold water
1 large clove **Garlic**, minced
1 tablespoon **Olive Oil**
1 cup **Crushed Pineapple**, packed in water or natural juices, well-drained (save juice for dressing)

1. Heat a large frying pan or wok; add oil. Sauté onions and garlic for 2-3 minutes until onions begin to soften.

2. Add red peppers and sauté a few minutes more, then add pork pieces. Stir until pork loses its raw appearance. Add cabbage and continue stirring until cabbage begins to soften.

3. Add Southeast Asian Sesame Pineapple dressing, crushed pineapple, and water chestnuts, and stir until both are heated through.

4. Stir arrowroot into cold water until smooth paste forms. Stir directly into boiling liquid, then distribute through entire mixture. Heat until sauce thickens.

1 serving = 421 kcal; 27g protein; 37g carbohydrate (6g fiber); 16.6g fat (3g saturated)

SOUTHEAST ASIAN PINEAPPLE SESAME DRESSING

Makes ¾ cup

From Moosewood Restaurant Low-Fat Favorites. *This makes a particularly good flavorful and slightly sweet marinade for vegetables, or it can be used to dress up fish, chicken, or tempeh.*

¼ cup **Unsweetened Crushed Pineapple**
1 tablespoon **Light Miso** (such as barley, chickpea, shiro)
1 tablespoon **Tamari**
1 tablespoon **Rice Vinegar**
1 tablespoon **Sesame Oil**
1 clove **Garlic**
¼ cup **Water or Unsweetened Pineapple Juice**

Place all ingredients in blender or food processor and purée until smooth.

3 tablespoons = 59 kcal; 1g protein; 5g carbohydrate; 3.7g unsaturated fat

GLAZED PORK AND APPLE SAUTE
Serves 4

1 pound **Pork Tenderloin** or other lean cut
2 teaspoons **Olive Oil**
1 tablespoon **Butter**
1 teaspoon **Arrowroot**
⅔ cup **Apple Juice**
2 tablespoons **Apple Juice**
¼ cup **Dry Sherry** (optional)
¼ teaspoon **White Pepper**
½ cup plain low-fat **Yogurt**
2 medium **Apples**, pared, cored, and cut into ¼-inch slices
½ cup **Onion**, diced

1. Slice pork into thin strips or rounds. Sauté in olive oil about 4 minutes until cooked through. Remove to a plate.

2. Add butter to the skillet. Sauté diced onion 2-3 minutes until it softens. Add apple slices and continue to sauté 3-4 minutes.

3. Add ⅔ cup apple juice and sherry and bring to boil. Reduce heat and add pork strips. Simmer 2 minutes.

4. While pork is simmering, combine arrowroot with 2 tablespoons apple juice until completely dissolved. Pour into skillet and stir until mixture thickens and become clear. Season with white pepper.

5. Stir in the yogurt just before serving and simmer gently to heat yogurt without boiling.

1 serving = 292 kcal; 27g protein; 20g carbohydrate (2g fiber); 11.1g fat (4g saturated)

ROAST BEEF, TURKEY, OR HAM ROLL-UPS

If you have no health problems that limit your use of dairy, this filling is great for a quick, low-carb snack that will hold you. It is easy for packed lunches or when you need food for a car or plane trip. I either roll up the filling in sliced deli meats or serve it with scoopers of celery sticks or sweet red bell peppers.

Sliced Deli Roast Beef or Turkey (no MSG, nitrates, or sugar)
1 recipe **Cream Cheese Spread** (below)

Figure on 1-2 rolls for a snack, 3-4 for a meal. Use a 1-ounce slice of lean roast beef, turkey, or ham per roll.

Spread a rounded tablespoon of spread on a slice of meat. Roll up the meat. If desired, roll up with a dill pickle spear, a cucumber stick, or red bell pepper stick tucked inside. Or pack along on the outside.

1 roast beef roll = 63 kcal; 6g protein; 1g carbohydrate; 3.3 g fat (2g saturated)
1 ham roll = 83 kcal; 9g protein; 2g carbohydrate; 5.1g fat (2g saturated)
1 turkey roll = 56 kcal; 5g protein; 1g carbohydrate; 2.6g fat (1g saturated)

CREAM CHEESE FILLING

Makes 10 servings of about 2 tablespoons

8 ounces **Neufchatel** (a light cream cheese), softened
2 **Scallions**, finely chopped
2 stalks **Celery**, finely chopped
6 **Black or Green Olives**, chopped
⅔ cup chopped, cooked **Spinach or Kale**, squeezed dry
    (frozen spinach works well)
Pinch of **Cayenne** or ground **Chipotle Pepper** (optional)

1. In a bowl, work Neufchatel around with back of spoon to break it up.

2. Add scallions, celery, spinach, or kale and mix until combined.

3. Add olives and mix just long enough to evenly distribute. Refrigerate.

2 tablespoons filling = 68 kcal; 1g protein; 2g carbohydrate; 5.1 g fat (3g saturated)

SEAFOOD

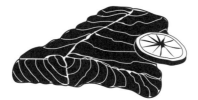

GINGER SALMON

Serves 4

A simple and delicious way to get your Omega 3 fats!

1½ pounds **Salmon Steak or Fillet**, rinsed and dried
2 teaspoons **Olive or Peanut Oil**
1 tablespoon grated fresh **Ginger Root**
¼ cup **Mirin***
2 tablespoons **Tamari or Soy Sauce**
1 **Green Onion**, sliced fine

1. Heat heavy skillet; when hot, add olive oil, then salmon. Sauté salmon 2 minutes a side for fillet or 3 minutes a side for steak. While fish cooks, combine all remaining ingredients except green onion in a bowl.

2. Pour sauce over fish; cover and simmer 1 minute more per side or until fish flakes easily.

3. Garnish with green onion.

1 serving = 296 kcal; 33g protein; 10g carbohydrate; 12.5g unsaturated fat

*All the carbohydrates in this recipe come from the mirin, a sweetened rice wine. If you want to lower the carb count to almost nothing, or if you prefer to avoid the alcohol, replace the mirin with rice vinegar and add a couple drops of stevia to provide the sweetness of the mirin.

SIMPLE POACHED SALMON
Serves 4

1¼ - 1½ pounds **Salmon (Fillet or Steak)**
3 cloves **Garlic**, sliced
1 **Lemon**, thinly sliced
1 stalk of **Celery**, cut in half
5 sprigs fresh **Dill** or 1 teaspoon dried dill
10 **Black Peppercorns** or 1 teaspoon ground black pepper
¼ teaspoon **Salt**

1. In large skillet add water to a ¾-inch depth. Add all ingredients except salmon. Bring to a boil, reduce heat, cover, and simmer 5 minutes.

2. Add salmon. Poach uncovered until cooked through, 2-3 minutes per side for fillet, 4-5 minutes per side for steak

1 serving = 206 kcal; 28g protein; 9.2g unsaturated fat

BAKED SCROD WITH GINGER PESTO
Serves 4

1¼ pounds **Scrod, Cod**, or **Halibut,** rinsed and dried
Salt and Pepper to taste
Olive Oil Spray
4 tablespoons plus 4 teaspoons **Ginger Pesto** (below)

1.   Lightly salt and pepper fish. Divide into 4 portions. Spray a baking pan with olive oil and place fish in pan. Spread 1 teaspoon of ginger pesto thinly over each piece of fish. Bake at 350° for 20 minutes or until fish begins to flake easily with a fork.

2.   Spread 1 tablespoon ginger pesto over each piece of fish.

1 serving = 221 kcal; 28g protein; 10.4g fat (1 saturated)

GINGER PESTO
Makes 1 cup
I found a version of this really unusual pesto on the Web, made a few adjustments, and voila! The possibilities are endless!

¼ cup packed, minced, fresh **Cilantro** (mince first, then pack)
¼ cup minced **Scallions**
¼ cup minced, peeled **Ginger Root** (peel, mince, measure)
½ cup **Macadamia Nuts**, chopped (measure, chop)
⅛ teaspoon **White Pepper**
¼ teaspoon **Salt** (or to taste)
½ cup **Walnut Oil**

1 tablespoon = 87 kcal; 9.4g fat (1 saturated)

Variation: Mix leftover pesto with plain, low-fat yogurt in a ratio of 2:1, yogurt to pesto. Use this as a vegetable dip or as an alternative to mayonnaise in cold fish salad, with sliced turkey or cold chicken.

2 tablespoons = 67 kcal; 1g carbohydrate; 6.7g unsaturated fat

---

SALMON CAKES
WITH HORSERADISH DRESSING
Serves 4

1 can **Pink, Red, or Sockeye Salmon** (14½ ounces)
1 **Egg**
1 **Egg White** or reconstituted powdered white
2 tablespoons **Prepared Horseradish**
1½ teaspoons dried **Dill Weed** or 2 tablespoons fresh
2 teaspoons finely chopped **Walnuts**
¼ teaspoons **Salt** or to taste
1½ tablespoons **Olive Oil**

Dressing:
4 teaspoons **Mayonnaise**
4 tablespoons **Prepared Horseradish**
1 teaspoon **Dill Weed**

1. Drain salmon. Remove skin and visible bones.* Mix all ingredients except oil in small bowl until thoroughly blended.

2. Run hands under cold water. Form salmon mixture into 4 patties. You may make these ahead and refrigerate at this point if desired.

3. Heat cast iron or heavy bottomed skillet. Add olive oil and spread around. Fry the salmon cakes 3-4 minutes per side until browned.

4. While salmon cakes cook, combine dressing ingredients and mix well. Top each patty with ¼ of the dressing.

1 serving = 288 kcal; 25g protein; 2g carbohydrate; 18.3g fat (2g saturated)

*The tiny bones in canned salmon are quite soft and provide an excellent source of calcium. I generally only remove the larger pieces; the rest will mash up nicely.

CREAMY SEAFOOD CHOWDER

Makes 2 quarts

This is wonderfully tasty nondairy chowder. No one you serve it to will notice that it's nondairy.

1½ cups chopped **Onion**
1 tablespoon **Olive Oil**
1 tablespoon **Arrowroot** or **Flour**
3 cups **Fish Stock** (or Chicken Stock)
2 cups peeled, seeded **Cucumber** (1 large)
1 12-ounce package **Silken Tofu***, drained
4 teaspoons fresh **Lemon Juice**
2 tablespoons minced fresh **Dill** or 1½ teaspoons dried
½ pound **Bay Scallops**, rinsed well
½ pound **Salmon Fillet,** skin removed
½ pound **Whitefish, Cod, or Halibut** (or any other mild fish)
Salt and Pepper to taste

1. In a soup pot, sauté the onion in olive oil over low heat, stirring, for several minutes. If using flour, add the flour and stir well for one minute. If using arrowroot, add per instructions in step 4.

2. Stir in the broth, bring to a boil, then turn down heat and simmer, being careful thickened soup doesn't stick to pot bottom.

3. In a blender, purée tofu, cucumber, lemon juice until smooth. Set aside.

4. Cut up fish into 1-inch pieces and add fish and scallops to simmering broth. Cook for 3-4 minutes until fish is firm. If using arrowroot, dissolve in 1-2 tablespoons cold water and stir until smooth. Add to soup and bring to boil until broth thickens. Turn down heat to low. Stir in tofu mixture, dill, salt, and pepper to taste and heat through, but don't boil.

1 cup serving = 191 kcal; 24g protein; 7g carbohydrate; 7g unsaturated fat

---

*Although I recommend very limited use of tofu, I do use it occasionally when I need to create a dairyless alternative to a standard recipe. Silken tofu has a custard-like consistency and is sold in aseptic packs in most grocery store.

CAJUN COD
Serves 4

1½ pounds **Cod or Whitefish**
1½ teaspoons **Onion Powder**
1 tablespoon **Chili Powder**
¼ teaspoon **Salt**
½ teaspoon **Black Pepper**
Pinch **Cayenne Pepper** (optional)
¾ cup low-fat **Sour Cream**
3 tablespoons **Scallions**
1 large **Cucumber**, peeled, seeded, and diced

1. Preheat broiler or grill. Combine spices in a bowl. Sprinkle on both sides of fish.

2. Grill or broil 4-5 minutes per side for cod, 2-3 for whitefish or until fish flakes easily.

3. Combine sour cream, cucumbers, and scallions in a bowl. Serve on top of or alongside of fish.

1 serving = 197 kcal; 32g protein; 6g carbohydrate; 4.2g fat (1g saturated)

LEMON PEPPER COD

Serves 4

1½ pounds **Cod**
1 tablespoon plus 1 teaspoon **Olive Oil**
¼ teaspoon **Lemon Pepper**

1. Rinse fish and pat dry. Brush with oil on both sides. Sprinkle with lemon pepper.

2. Bake at 375° for 10-12 minutes, turning halfway through.

1 serving = 156 kcal; 25g protein; 5.5g unsaturated fat

SALMON AND SCALLOP KABOBS WITH ASIAN MARINADE

Serves 4

The marinade used in this recipe is a good one to keep on hand for putting together an elegant but easy meal. This kabob can be done with chicken or tempeh as well, and is an easy summertime dinner that needs only a green vegetable to round it out.

¾ pound **Salmon fillet**
½ pound large **Sea Scallops** (9 or 10)
1 **Sweet Red Bell Pepper**
8 thick **Scallions**
½ cup **Asian Marinade** (page 268)
4 cups **Mung Bean Sprouts,** left raw
½ cup grated **Carrot**
4 wooden **skewers,** soaked 5 minutes in water

1. Rinse fish and scallops and pat dry. Cut salmon into cubes to match the size of scallops. Remove skin if desired.

2. Place in nonreactive pan or bowl and gently toss with marinade.

3. Seed pepper and cut into 1-inch squares. Wash and trim scallions and cut thick white portion into 1-inch lengths. Add both to marinade mixture. Let sit 15 minutes.

4. Place fish and vegetables on the 4 skewers, alternating items.

5. Place on hot grill for 2-3 minutes a side. While fish is grilling, bring remaining marinade to a boil to use at table, if desired.*

6. Remove fish and vegetables from the skewer. Serve on a bed of mung sprouts and grated carrot.

1 serving = 283 kcal; 30g protein; 17g carbohydrate (4g fiber); 10.5g unsaturated fat

---

***Important Safety Note**: Never use a marinade after it has had raw meat or fish in it, unless you either boil it first or baste it on while the food is cooking.*

TUNA WALDORF SALAD

Serves 2

Tuna is such a great source of lean protein, but plain tuna can get old fast. Try this version for a protein-packed, new twist. This is adapted from a favorite of mine from my colleague Rachel Albert-Matesz of Next Generation Nutrition.

2 6-ounce cans **Tuna**, water-packed, drained
1½ **Granny Smith** or other tart apple, seeded and chopped
½ cup **Sweet Onion**, minced
1½ **Celery** stalks, diced
2 tablespoons plus 2 teaspoons chopped toasted **Walnuts** (page 281)
4 teaspoons **Mayonnaise**
    (or 3 tablespoons Lemon Miso Tahini dressing-page 264)
2 tablespoons plain, low-fat **Yogurt** (leave out if using Lemon Miso Tahini dressing)
4 cups mixed **Salad Greens** or torn **Lettuce**

1. Combine all ingredients except salad greens.

2. Serve tuna on top of bed of greens.

1 serving = 320 kcal; 35g protein; 22g carbohydrate (6g fiber); 10.5g fat (1g saturated)

Variation: Try using cooked, white meat turkey in place of tuna.

TUNA IN RED PEPPER BOATS
Serves 1 or 2

1 6-ounce can **Albacore Tuna,** water-packed, drained (will yield 4 ounces)
1 **Sweet Red Bell Pepper**
1 tablespoon **Mayonnaise** (use reduced fat only if it contains no sugar)
2 tablespoons finely chopped **Celery**
2 tablespoons minced **Scallions**
1 teaspoon dried **Dill Weed**
Salt and Pepper to taste
2 tablespoons **Dill Pickle Relish** (no sugar added) if desired
    (or use chopped **Dill Pickle**)
1 ounce **Smoked Mozzarella or Cheese of Choice**, in thin slices

1. Cut the pepper in half and remove seeds and membranes. Place face down in a small oven-proof pan and put under broiler for 5-8 minutes until skin begin to soften and bubble. Turn over once and let underside broil for 2-3 minutes.

2. While pepper is broiling, drain tuna and mix with remaining ingredients except for the cheese.

3. Stuff tuna into broiled pepper halves; top each half with cheese. Put back under broiler until cheese starts to melt and becomes brown and bubbly.

2 pepper boat halves = 303 kcal; 33g protein; 7g carbohydrate (2g fiber); 14.5g fat (2g saturated)

SWEET TREATS

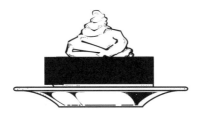

STRAWBERRY CRANBERRY TOPPING

Makes 3¾ cups

This naturally sweetened topping is delightful mixed with plain yogurt or used as a topping for Whey Better Pancakes (page256) or Sprouted French Toast (page258)

3 cups frozen **Strawberries**
1 cup fresh **Cranberries**
¾ cup **Raisins**
Stevia Liquid to taste

1. Put all the fruit in medium-sized pot. Bring to a boil, then turn heat down to a simmer.

2. Cover and simmer until raisins are swelled and cranberries have popped.

3. Add stevia to taste.

¼ cup = 41 kcal; 11g carbohydrate (1g fiber); .1g unsaturated fat

JUDY'S YOGURT SUNDAE

This makes a wonderful after-school snack for kids or a mid-afternoon energy booster for anyone. It also packs well for a lunch or road trip.

½ cup plain low-fat **Yogurt**
¼ cup **Strawberry Cranberry Topping**
1 tablespoon ground **Flax Meal**
⅔ ounce **Vanilla Whey Protein Powder** (stevia sweetened)

Stir protein powder into yogurt until well-blended.
Add topping and stir to blend. Sprinkle flax meal on top.

1 serving = 206 kcal; 21g protein; 22g carbohydrate (3g fiber); 4.9g fat (1g saturated)

Note: If mixture has a chance to sit for a while, the protein powder absorbs moisture from the yogurt, giving it the consistency of pudding.

FROZEN CAPPUCCINO LATTÉ

Serves 1

This is my very favorite sweet treat. I sometimes have it for breakfast if I want to be extra nice to myself for having to get to work early and take breakfast to my desk.

⅓ medium frozen **Banana** (about 2¾ inches long)
1 ounce **Vanilla Whey Protein Powder** (1 scoop)
⅔ cup **Water**
⅔ teaspoon **Coffee Extract**
⅔ teaspoon **Cinnamon** or to taste
1 teaspoon **Flaxseed Oil**
4 **ice cubes**

1. For ease in blending, place ice cubes in plastic bag and smash with hammer to partially crush.

2. Place all ingredients in blender and blend on high speed until smooth and creamy.

1 serving = 174 kcal; 23g protein; 10g carbohydrate (1g fiber); 5.7g unsaturated fat

---

Variation: Need a quick but nourishing lunch, or a breakfast that carries you a little longer? Make this a little more substantial by replacing the water with 2% milk and adding an extra teaspoon of flax oil.

1 serving = 325 kcal; 28g protein; 18g carbohydrate (1g fiber); 18.8g fat (2g saturated)

PROTEIN NUT BUTTER DELIGHT

Makes 2 cups

My friend and colleague, Rachel Albert-Matesz, came up with this amazing combination which makes a fabulous snack for kids and adults. The protein powder and water help "dilute" the fat content of the nut butter.

½ cup plus 2 tablespoons **Filtered Water**
½ cup **Nut Butter** (almond, cashew, peanut, hazelnut)
1 cup **Vanilla Whey Protein Powder**
Pinch **Salt**

1.   Bring the water to a boil with a pinch of salt, then turn off heat.

2.   Add nut butter and combine with spoon until smooth and free of lumps.

3.   Stir in whey protein powder and mix until smooth and creamy.

4.   Refrigerate spread. Will keep about 2 weeks if it lasts that long! Serve with fruit.

2 tablespoons = 104 kcal; 13g protein; 3g carbohydrate (1g fiber); 4.2 g unsaturated fat
With ½ medium apple = 144 kcal; 14g carbohydrate (3g fiber); 5g unsaturated fat

---

Variations: Experiment by adding ½ teaspoon or so of different flavored extracts. One combination I've tried and is a hit in my cooking classes is butterscotch extract with almond butter. Also, try using chocolate whey protein if you're a chocolate fan.

BANANA JEWELS
Makes 2 dozen

This is a great way to give your kids (or yourself) a sweet treat that doesn't have added sugar and is reasonably low in refined, high-glycemic flour. They're fairly moist, so if you have any left after a few days, pop 'em in the fridge. These freeze well too.

1¼ cups **Rolled Oats** (not quick-cooking)
½ cup **Oat, Millet or Kamut Flour**
½ teaspoon **Salt**
¼ teaspoon **Baking Soda**
Dash or 2 **Ground Cinnamon**
2 tablespoons **Chopped Raisins**
2 tablespoons **Chopped Nuts** (optional)
1 cup mashed **Ripe Banana**
6 tablespoons **Walnut Oil**

1.   Preheat oven to 350°. Mix all dry ingredients together.

2.   In separate bowl blend bananas and oil, then add to dry ingredients and mix well.

3.   Drop by heaping teaspoons on ungreased cookie sheet. Bake for 10-15 minutes

1 cookie = 81 kcal; 1g protein; 9g carbohydrate (.5g fiber); 4.3g unsaturated fat

APRICOT NUT ROLLS
Makes 12

These little gems are fairly calorie- and carbohydrate-dense for their size, so save them for a special occasion or a very active day.

10 **Dried Apricot Halves** (unsulfured)*
2½ tablespoons **Pine Nuts**
3 tablespoons **Walnuts**
1 rounded tablespoon **Vanilla Whey Protein Powder** (see page 250)
1 tablespoon **Orange Juice**
Coconut or Pecan Meal for rolling

1. Chop up apricot halves into smaller pieces. Place all ingredients except coconut or pecan meal in food processor. Mix until you have a dough-like ball.

2. Run hands under cold water to prevent dough from sticking. Pinch a teaspoon or so of dough and roll into small ball or cylinder. Roll in pecan meal or coconut. Repeat with remaining dough.

3. These are best if allowed to sit in refrigerator for at least four hours.

1 roll = 45 kcal; 2g protein; 18g carbohydrate (2g fiber); 2.2g unsaturated fat (rolled in coconut)

---

*Often dried fruit is preserved with sulfur compounds called sulfites. These agents are used to prevent spoilage and discoloration in dried fruit, in wine, on salad bars, and many other places. Many people suffer allergic reactions to sulfites, primarily affecting the respiratory system. One out of ten asthmatics is likely to have such a reaction, which can be so extreme as to be fatal. Look for "sulfite-free" dried fruits when you shop.

CAROB FUDGIES

Makes 13 balls

These delightful energy balls make a sweet treat that won't send your blood sugar and you on a roller coaster ride. If eating chocolate is a problem for you, these have a fudgy taste that is different but still satisfies. These are from The Fat Burning Diet *by Jay Robb.*

3 tablespoons **Carob Powder**

3 1-ounce scoops **Vanilla Whey Protein Powder** (see page 250)

1½ tablespoons unrefined **Hazelnut, Walnut, Pistachio, or Flaxseed Oil**

¼ cup raw or lightly toasted **Cashews, Walnuts, Hazelnuts, Almonds, or Pecans**

2-4 tablespoons seedless **Raisins**, chopped
    (vary according to how sweet you want it)

2 teaspoons **Rice Bran or Apple Fiber**

¾ teaspoon of either ground **nutmeg, ginger, or cinnamon** (optional)

Filtered Water as needed to moisten (2-4 tablespoons)

Shredded Coconut to roll balls in (optional)

1. Mix all dry ingredients together in bowl with a fork, until well blended.

2. Add the oil and continue blending until well distributed.

3. Add water a little at a time and stir until mixture is moist but stiff enough to roll into balls.

4. Moisten hands with cold water. Roll mixture into 13 walnut-sized balls. If you like, roll balls to coat with shredded coconut. Refrigerate at least 1 hour before serving.

1 ball = 66 kcal; 5g protein; 5g carbohydrate; 3g unsaturated fat

---

Variation: Substitute chocolate-flavored whey protein powder for vanilla. If you are lactose-intolerant or avoid dairy for any reason, try Jay Robb® Egg White Protein Powder. You will need to add a bit of stevia to the recipe because the egg white powder is not as sweet as the whey powder. Egg White Protein available at **www.jayrobb.com**.

BUTTERSCOTCH PUDDING

Serves 6

This healthy version tastes so much better than the stuff out of the box! Topped with a dollop of whipped cream, it makes a very special dessert. Serve it with a meal that has been light in carbohydrates.

2 cup cooked mashed **Yams** (Red Garnet gives sweetest flavor)*
1 cup original-flavored **Amasake****
1 Egg
1 ounce scoop **Vanilla Whey Protein Powder** (see page 250)
1½ teaspoons natural **Butterscotch Flavoring**
2-4 drops **Stevia Liquid**

1. Blend all ingredients in blender or food processor until very smooth.

2. Pour in baking dish or individual ramekins. Bake at 350° for 30 minutes or until custard is set and the top is golden brown. Can serve warm or chilled.

1 serving = 133 kcal; 6g protein; 22g carbohydrate (1g fiber); 1.7g unsaturated fat

---

*Red Garnet is the queen of yams as far as I'm concerned. They have the sweetest, smoothest flavor and can be used creatively in many recipes, a plus when you're trying to get more vegetables in your kids. To bake yams, scrub, wrap in foil and bake at 400° for an hour or until very soft. If yams are organic, the soft peel can be eaten for extra nutrients. Red Garnets are reddish purple, just like their namesake, and are typically longer and narrower than a traditional yam or sweet potato.

** Amasake is a thick, very sweet liquid made from fermenting brown rice. Its sweetness is naturally occurring and fermenting the rice makes it a very digestible, nutritionally available food. However, it should be used sparingly, because even though its sweetness is natural, it still affects blood sugar levels.

CHOCOLATE MOUSSE

Serves 6

This light dessert will make your taste buds—not your blood sugar—soar.

⅔ cup **Boiling Water**
2 teaspoons **Unflavored Gelatin**
⅔ cup **Lite Coconut Milk**
2 tablespoons **Unsweetened Cocoa**
2 tablespoons **Cashew Butter**
5 tablespoons **Chocolate Whey Protein Powder** (see page 250)
15 drops **Stevia Liquid**
½ teaspoon **Coffee Extract** (may substitute vanilla)
8 **Ice Cubes**, crushed

1. Place boiling water first, then gelatin in blender, and whip for several minutes. While this is blending, assemble other ingredients. Place ice cubes in plastic bag and use hammer to crush into smaller pieces.

2. Add all remaining ingredients to blender except ice. Blend for a minute or until well combined.

3. Add crushed ice and blend until completely smooth. Pour into individual dishes and chill.

1 serving = 133 kcal; 9g protein; 5g carbohydrate; 4.4g unsaturated fat

BERRY DELICIOUS SORBET
Serves 2

2 cups frozen **Strawberries, Raspberries, or Mixed Berries**
2 tablespoons plain low-fat **Yogurt**
¼ cup **Milk**
2 drops **Stevia Liquid** or to taste
¼ teaspoon **Vanilla Extract**
2 tablespoons **Chopped Nuts**
Fresh Berries (if available, for garnish)

1. Five minutes before serving, remove fruit from freezer to soften slightly.

2. When ready to serve, place all ingredients in food processor. Purée until smooth.

3. Serve immediately, garnished with chopped nuts and berries.

1 serving = 136 kcal; 3g protein; 18g carbohydrate (6g fiber); 6.4g unsaturated fat

---

Variations: Try making this with different fruit or combinations, such as mango, mango and peach, strawberry and banana, kiwi, pineapple. Remember that fruits such as banana or mango have very high sugar contents and a 1-cup serving would yield more sugar than the same amount of berries. Refer to the block chart on pages 84-87 to help you make appropriate choices for your needs.

BANANA SCREAMS

Serves 3

From Charles Hunt's Diet Evolution *(with a slight name change!)*

1 medium **Banana** (8-9 inches long)
1 tablespoon plus 1½ teaspoons **Smooth Peanut Butter**
⅓ cup **Shredded Coconut** (unsweetened)

1. For easier handling, peel and cut banana in half crosswise. Spread ½ the peanut butter in a thin layer over the outside of each banana half.

2. Place coconut in a shallow bowl. Slice the banana into ½-inch slices, allowing them to drop into the coconut. Roll each slice to coat with coconut on all surfaces.

3. Put the slices on a plate. Place in freezer for several hours until frozen. Remove frozen slices from plate and store in sealed container.

1 serving = 113 kcal; 2g protein; 8g carbohydrate; 7.7g fat (3g saturated)

APPLE CRANBERRY FRUIT COMPOTE

Serves 12

A creation of kitchen wizard and cookbook author, Rachel Albert-Matesz

4-5 medium **Apples**
2 cups fresh **Cranberries** (frozen will work, too, out of season)
1 cup **Raisins**
1 12-ounce bag frozen **Strawberries or Mixed Berries**
¼ cup **Water**
Stevia Liquid to taste

1. Wash, core, and slice apples into large, wide pot. Layer cranberries, frozen berries, and raisins on top. Add ¼ cup water.

2. Cover and bring to a boil. Reduce to a simmer and cook for about 25-30 minutes until apples are tender and cranberries have popped.

3. Remove from heat. Stir to mix fruit. Add stevia to bring to desired level of sweetness.

4. When compote has cooled some, spoon into quart jars for storing. Compote will thicken as it cools.

½ **cup serving** = 71 kcal; 20g carbohydrate (2g fiber); 0.3 grams unsaturated fat

---

Because this dessert contains no protein and virtually no fat, it is best eaten with some of both to keep blood sugar balanced. Some people may be able to easily assimilate the 20g of carbohydrate, but anyone with sensitivity to carbohydrates will not. Try using it in the following ways:

Sweeten plain yogurt
Use as topping for Whey Better Pancakes
Serve as condiment for poultry or pork
Serve as dessert with 1 or 2 tablespoons of cream or half-and-half and 1 tablespoon of unsweetened granola topping

PUMPKIN SOUFFLÉ

Serves 5

These soufflés have a wonderful texture and mixture of spices reminiscent of traditional New England Indian Pudding. This makes a nice ending to a Thanksgiving meal or a treat for a cool fall or winter evening.

1½ cups **Pumpkin Purée**
2 tablespoons low-fat **Sour Cream**
¼ teaspoon grated **Nutmeg**
Pinch **Allspice**
Pinch **Cinnamon**
¾ teaspoon **Natural Maple Flavoring**
½ teaspoon **Natural Vanilla Extract**
15 drops **Stevia Liquid**
1 teaspoon **Trutina®**
Pinch freshly ground **Pepper**
5 **Egg Whites**
½ cup **Whipping Cream**
½ cup **Pecans,** lightly toasted and chopped (see page 281)

1. Preheat oven to 425°. In large bowl, blend pumpkin, maple flavor, low-fat sour cream, spices, and pepper.

2. In another large bowl, beat egg whites until stiff but not dry. Gently fold about ¼ of whites into the pumpkin mixture, then fold in remaining whites.

3. Gently pour into individual soufflé dishes or custard cups; smooth tops.

4. Bake until soufflé has puffed, 18-20 minutes. While soufflé bakes, toast pecans in dry frying pan over low heat for several minutes, until fragrant.

5. Serve soufflé warm with whipped cream and pecans.

1 serving = 161 kcal; 5g protein; 8g carbohydrate (2g fiber); 12.5g fat (5g saturated)

Variation: Maple Whipped Cream
1 cup **Heavy Whipping Cream,** beat until stiff. Then add
¾ teaspoon **Natural Maple Flavor**
½ teaspoon **Trutina®** or **Stevia Liquid** to taste (2-3 drops)

NUTRITION MAGICIAN'S FUDGE

Serves 12

Protein never tasted so good! Bring this, confidently, anywhere people scoff at healthful food!

1 square unsweetened **Baking Chocolate**
2 tablespoons **Butter**
2 tablespoons **Half-and-Half**
½ cup **Chocolate Whey Protein Powder**
   (or use **Vanilla Whey Protein Powder** with 1 tablespoon **Unsweetened Cocoa**)
¼ cup **Almonds,** toasted
1 tablespoon **Flaxseed Oil**
1 tablespoon **Water**

1. In top of double boiler, melt chocolate and butter. While this is happening, toast almonds over medium heat for several minutes in dry frying pan, shaking frequently. Chop when toasted.

2. Remove from heat; add half-and-half and flaxseed oil. Stir to incorporate until mixture thickens slightly. Stir in protein powder until well-mixed. Add chopped almonds.

3. Add water gradually only if mixture isn't binding together—amount will vary with humidity. Do not use entire tablespoon right away, as you may not need all. Use just enough water to bind; you don't want excess liquid in bottom of pan.

4. Press into pan and spread into 5-inch x 7-inch rectangle. Refrigerate several hours, then cut into 12 pieces.

1 piece = 110 kcal: 12g protein; 3g carbohydrate; 6g fat (1g saturated)

GLOSSARY
OF FOOD AND
INGREDIENTS

Arrowroot is a plant starch used for thickening. Its name comes from *Aru Root* because it was said to be an antidote to poison arrows used by the Aruac Indians of South America. Arrowroot is an alternative to using corn-based cornstarch in cooking. It must first be dissolved in cold water, then added to hot liquid. Arrowroot won't stay in solution in cold water, so you must stir it well just before adding to the liquid that you want thickened.

Amasake is a thick, very sweet liquid made from fermenting brown rice. Its sweetness is naturally occurring and fermenting the rice makes it a very digestible, nutritionally available food. However, it should be used sparingly, because even though its sweetness is natural, it still affects blood-sugar levels. While it is sold as a beverage to drink as is, I don't recommend this because of the sugar content. Amasake is sold in health food stores in a refrigerator case and comes in several flavors. It keeps well in the freezer.

Baba Ghanouj is a Middle-Eastern dip made from mashed, roasted eggplant to which sesame butter (tahini), lemon juice, and seasonings are added. It makes a good dip for raw vegetables or can be eaten on whole-grain crackers. Many grocery stores now carry prepared baba ghanouj.

Bok Choy is one of several Chinese cabbages now commonly available. A great source of absorbable calcium, bok choy is delicious in salads raw, or added to stir-fry dishes. It has a fleshy, crisp, white, center rib with dark green leaves.

Brown Rice Vinegar will usually be found in stores that have a macrobiotic food section. Because it is made from brown rice, this vinegar is less acidic and has a milder taste than white, cider, or balsamic vinegars.

Carob Powder is a cocoa-like substance made from the carob bean. Although it looks like chocolate, it has a very different flavor but is often used by people who avoid chocolate for health reasons. It can substitute for cocoa in any recipe. Carob is naturally sweet, unlike cocoa, so products made from carob typically have fewer sweeteners added to them. Carob also does not contain caffeine.

Chipotle Chili is a type of pepper that has been dried and smoked. Along with adding some heat to a dish as any other hot pepper would, it also gives the same kind of smoky flavor that liquid smoke or cooking with a ham hock gives. Soak chipotle chilies in hot water for about ten minutes before adding to a recipe. You do not need to remove the seeds as is often done with other chili peppers.

Coconut Milk is a thick liquid made from coconut meat. It is high in lauric acid, healthy fat that is both antiviral and antibacterial. Although a saturated fat, it is well digested and a healthful addition to the diet. Lauric acid is also a major component of mothers' breast milk. Look for pure coconut milk with no additives.

Daikon Radish looks like a very long, fat, white carrot. It is a mild-tasting radish that gets even milder with cooking. In Chinese medicine, daikon radish has a number of healing properties, including liver detoxification and clearing mucous from the lungs. It is delicious raw, steamed, or stir-fried.

Delicata and Dumpling Squashes are too less well-known but delicious varieties of winter squash. They both have a beige skin with green stripes. Delicata is oblong shaped, and dumpling, like its name suggests, is short, squat, and round. They can either be baked or steamed after the seeds inside have been removed.

Fennel is commonly known as a spice with a licorice flavor, similar to anise. But it is also a vegetable frequently used in Italian cooking. Fennel has a large bulbous end with celery-like stalks coming out of it. Fennel can be eaten raw in salads or used for dipping; when eaten raw it has a more pronounced licorice flavor. It can also be braised, baked, or grilled.

Fish Sauce is a mainstay flavoring used in Thai, Vietnamese, and Cambodian cooking, analogous to soy sauce in Chinese cooking. It does not give a flavor to most dishes that one would identify as fish, although the plain sauce itself smells fishy. Fish sauce is an aged product made from fresh fish.

Hokkaido Squash, also known as Kabucha or Japanese Pumpkin, is dark green and looks somewhat like a flattened pumpkin. It has the highest sugar content of any squash. It is similar to buttercup squash but has a drier texture that crumbles if overcooked. The skin is also edible. Hokkaido can be prepared like any winter squash—it is delicious baked. Its naturally sweet properties make it a satisfying food for people who are trying to limit their intake of concentrated sweeteners.

Hummus is the well-known Middle Eastern dip made from mashed chickpeas, sesame butter, lemon juice, garlic, and usually olive oil. Like its cousin baba ghanouj, hummus makes a good vegetable dip or whole grain cracker spread and can often be purchased prepared in grocery stores.

Jicama is crunchy, slightly sweet, and adds great texture and flavor to a salad. It looks like a flattened, wide turnip covered with a thick, light-brown skin. Choose jicamas that are small and firm, with few nicks or blemishes. Avoid larger ones, which are dry and flavorless. Jicama is a Mexican vegetable traditionally served with lime juice and a sprinkling of chili powder. It is also good cooked, retains its crunchiness, and is especially good in stir-fries.

Just Whites® is a brand of all-natural, powdered egg whites available in most grocery stores. It can be substituted easily for one or more whole eggs in omelets, scrambled eggs, or baked egg dishes such as quiche.

Lemon Grass is an essential ingredient to Southeast Asian cooking. The tough stalk is chopped and simmered in soups and the liquid of many other dishes to give a lemony scent and flavor. The stalk is too fibrous and tough to eat and is removed and discarded before serving.

Mirin is a type of Japanese sake or rice wine used in cooking. Because of its sweetness, it should be avoided or used judiciously by those who have to closely regulate their blood sugar.

Miso is a fermented bean paste that is used for soups in Japanese restaurants, but is also a delicious and healthful addition to dressings, marinades, and sauces. It is considered to be a medicinal food in macrobiotic cooking, one that helps maintain the balance of good bacteria within the gastrointestinal tract. Miso comes in many flavors and varieties; the darker ones are aged and stronger in flavor while lighter varieties are younger and sweeter. Look for it in a refrigerated case in your health food grocery store. For soups, add miso to liquid that has been brought to a boil then removed from the heat; do not boil it, as that will destroy the live bacteria. For each serving, mix a teaspoon to a tablespoon into a small amount of liquid until smooth paste results. Then add additional liquid. Store miso in the refrigerator.

Nappa Cabbage is a variety of Chinese cabbage suitable for salads, stir-fries, braising, or as an outer wrapper for a filling. These cabbages have a lighter-weight, more pliable leaf than traditional green cabbage, but leaves should not be at all limp. A head of nappa cabbage is usually from 8 to 12 inches tall and about 6 inches in diameter.

Neufchatel Cheese is a lower-fat version of cream cheese that substitutes easily in any recipe calling for cream cheese, including cheese cake. It is sometimes sold in packaging labeled as low-fat or light cream cheese, but should indicate somewhere on the packaging that it is Neufchatel.

Quinoa (pronounced keen-wa) is an ancient South American grain considered sacred by the Incas and recently rediscovered in North America. Compared to other grains and vegetables, it is high in protein, calcium, and iron and in ancient cultures was considered an ideal food for pregnant and nursing women. It looks like a cross between millet and sesame seeds. It is coated with a naturally occurring insect repellant called saponin and must be rinsed in warm water before cooking to remove the bitter taste of this coating. Quinoa is cooked with a ratio of 1½ cups liquid to one cup of grain for a drier, fluffier grain.

Sprouted Grain Bread is a flourless bread that looks and tastes like regular bread. Sprouted grain breads are very high in fiber and are digested as a vegetable rather than a starch. When wheat is milled into flour and refined, as is usually the case with bread, twenty-two vitamins and minerals are reduced by 40 to 70 percent, and only 7 percent of the fiber is left intact. This makes it a less nutritious food and causes elevations in blood sugar, which are unhealthy. Sprouting creates enzymes and develops amino acids, which aid digestion, and also increases the protein content of the bread. Sprouted grain bread is available in many varieties. If you cannot find sprouted grain breads at your local health food store, look online at **www.sunrisefds.com** or **www.oasisbreads.com**.

Stevia is an herbal sweetener for those who are concerned with health and blood-sugar regulation. See Chapter Ten for explanation and purchasing information.

Tahini is nut butter made from crushing sesame seeds. It makes a tasty addition to sauces and dips and is used often in Middle Eastern cooking.

Tamari is aged soy sauce that has no preservatives or flavorings (such as MSG) added to it. It can be purchased in a wheat-free variety (soy sauce contains wheat).

Tempeh is a pressed cake of cooked, fermented soybeans, often with the addition of various grains. It has a nutty flavor and absorbs the flavors of marinades and sauces very well. Because of the fermentation process, it does not have the disadvantage of blocking mineral absorption as many soy foods do. Tempeh is best prepared by lightly steaming for ten to fifteen minutes, then using it in whatever recipe you choose. The steaming mellows a strong flavor that some people find objectionable.

Umeboshi Plums are a salty, Japanese plum believed in Oriental medicine to have great medicinal value. They also add an unusual but delicious taste to food. The plums can be purchased whole or as a paste. Because they are highly salty, only a small amount is used at one time. Both plums and paste should be stored in refrigerator once opened, but they will last indefinitely if well-sealed. Find these in a health food store in the macrobiotic section.

Watercress is a peppery green that is a member of the same family as broccoli, cauliflower, brussel sprouts, and cabbage: the crucifers. It grows in and around water; will often be displayed in the produce section in a container of water. Look for something a little smaller than a bunch of parsley with more distinctly formed leaves. Watercress is frequently used in salads and soups. It is known for being high in vitamin C and other cancer-preventing phytochemicals.

Xanthan Gum, made from corn sugar, is used as a thickener and emulsifier in dairy products, salad dressings, and other foods. It provides a low-glycemic alternative to flour as a thickener and dissolves in either hot or cold liquids.

INDEX

ABOUT
THE AUTHOR

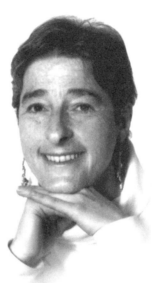

J udy Stone is a certified social worker with a Masters in Social Work from the University of Michigan, and was a practicing psychothererapist for over twenty years. She is certified in Bioenergetic Analysis, a body-mind psychotheraphy and has always included relationship-with-food issues and nutrition in her practice. She developed Feeding Your Whole Self, a program integrating nutrition, cooking skills and relationship-with-food-and-body issues in 1994, and also began publishing Eater's Digest-a print, then later an online-newsletter. In 1999 she decided to focus her practice exclusively on nutrition and pursued a certification in Comprehensive Nutrition through the American Academy of Nutrition. From her home in Ann Arbor, Michigan, Judy provides coaching and consultation to individuals throughout the United States as well as teaching, speaking, offering corporate wellness programs, and writing. In her spare time she plays ice hockey, loves experimenting in the kitchen, and enjoys her family. Judy can be contacted at 734-994-5549 or reached through her website, **www.taketwoapples.com**.

TAKE TWO APPLES
AND CALL ME IN THE MORNING
ORDER FORM

QTY.	Title	US Price	CN Price	Total
	Take Two Apples **and Call Me in the Morning**	**$21.95**	**$28.95**	
	Shipping and Handling Add $4.50 for orders in the US/Add $7.50 for Global Priority			
	Sales tax (WA state residents only, add 8.9%)			
	Total enclosed			

Telephone Orders:
Call 1-800-461-1931
Have your VISA or
MasterCard ready.

INTL. Telephone Orders:
Toll free 1-877-250-5500
Have your credit card ready.

Fax Orders:
425-398-1380
Fill out this order form and fax.

Postal Orders:
Hara Publishing
P.O. Box 19732
Seattle, WA 98109

E-mail Orders:
harapub@foxinternet.net

Method of Payment:

☐   Check or
Money Order

☐

☐ MasterCard

Expiration Date: _____

Card #: _____

Signature: _____

Name _____
Address _____
City _____ State ____ Zip _____
Phone ( ) _____ Fax ( ) _____

Quantity discounts are available.
Call 425-398-3679 for more information.
Thank you for your order!